What I Learned from Cancer

WHAT I
LEARNED
FROM
CANCER

Dennis Maione

Prompters to Life / Winnipeg

Book information available at
www.prompterstolife.com

Copyright © 2014 by Dennis Maione

All rights reserved under International and
Pan-American Copyright Conventions. Published
in Canada by Prompters to Life, Winnipeg.

Library and Archives Canada Cataloguing in Publication

Maione, Dennis, 1964-, author
What I learned from cancer / Dennis Maione.

Includes index.
Issued in print, electronic and audio formats.
ISBN 978-0-9937386-0-9 (bound). ISBN 978-0-9937386-1-6 (pbk.).
ISBN 978-0-9937386-3-0 (kindle). ISBN 978-0-9937386-4-7 (kobo).
ISBN 978-0-9937386-5-4 (ibook). ISBN 978-0-9937386-2-3 (audio)

1. Maione, Dennis, 1964-Health. 2. Cancer--Patients--Canada--
Biography. 3. Cancer--Psychological aspects. I. Title.

RC265.6.M334A3 2014   362.196'9940092   C2014-902909-8
                                              C2014-902910-1
                                              C2014-902911-X

Printed in Canada by Friesen Printers
Editing by WordsWorth Services (Debra Maione)
Graphics, Design, and Layout by Tiny Giant (Scott Hutchinson)

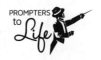

To Reg Litz, who showed me how to live and die well.

*"I have fought the good fight, I have finished
the race, I have kept the faith."*

Second Timothy 4:7 (NRSV)

Personal Acknowledgements

To Debra, my wife, my partner, my fellow-traveller in sickness and in health. Love and thanks are too little to show for the debt that I owe you.

To my children whom I love with all my heart:

Emma, who is put out because she is not mentioned in this book anywhere but here—know that I still love you more than any daughter could be loved.

Alexander, who shares too many things in common with me for us to always get along but enough that we will always share a common journey—may you learn, through my example, to revel in the joys of life and to persevere through its trials.

Noah, who got his own chapter in this book, much to the envy of others around him—I pray that you will approach all of your life with the courage you showed in the hospital.

To my dad, Albert Maione, and my step-mother, Lori Maione: thank you for your unending love to me and my family and for your support of this project.

To my mom, Pauline Margrette: thank you for your everlasting love and for giving me the gift of this story.

To Debra's parents, Henry and Eleonore Esau: thank you for ongoing support through this transition in our lives; the chance to do this and other projects means more to me than you will ever know.

To Angie, Jamie, Scott, Colleen, Len, Brian, and Rocio: well, I am supposed to thank all of my siblings, right? You have all encouraged and inspired me in innumerable ways.

To my relatives with Lynch syndrome: may we all live our lives to the fullest, regardless of the challenges that genetics have given to us.

To the special people in this story, the ones whom I mentioned by name and the ones whom I did not: my life would have been barren and oh-so-fleeting were it not for the contributions of each of you.

To the men in my book clubs over the years (John, Gerry, Reg, Roger, Murray, Dan, Kevin, Rick, Geoff, Gerald, and Peter): thanks for reminding me to read.

To Jake and the men and women in his writing group: thanks for encouraging me to write.

Special thanks to Gerry: thanks for sushi, Steven Pressfield, and for pushing me to believe in myself and in this book.

To God, who saved my body and my soul.

Kickstarter Acknowledgements

When I launched the Kickstarter project to fund the printing of this book, I held my breath and clicked "Publish." When I did so, I could not have imagined the outpouring of support that I received. I literally spent much of the first day in tears as I saw my family, friends, acquaintances, and strangers contribute to this project. This is community, and I thank each of you, regardless of the level of your contribution, for the faith you had in me when you pledged your support. For those of you who did not want to have your generosity acknowledged, I hope that you will feel sufficiently hidden in this crowd.

So, thank you to: Sheldon, John&Wendy, Chuck&Joanne, Rob&Colleen, Gerry&Karen, Scott&Jamie, Brandon&Kirsty, Steve&Carole, Pauline, Merle&Carol, Shelley, Heather, Len&Wanda, Jake, Sandy, Jenna, Brian&Elaine, Rod&Wendy, Rhonda, Mike&Wendy, Marcel&Leanne, Terri, Don&Carol, Mike, Cliff, Lori, Gary&Linda, Albert&Lori, Laura, Phil, Brad&Jan, Ellen, Andrew, Dave, Rod, Deborah, Phil, Zelma, Cheryl, Todd&Jan, Cordell&Amy, Jim, Judy, John, Jason, Marcel&Adria, Scott&Meredith, Rick, Brent, Faye, Rob, Denise, Cliff, Elaine, Kevin&Pam, Roberto, Teresa, Chris, Juanita, Hardy, Teresa, Robyn, Cheri, Rita, Rick&Shelly, Brian&Marliss, Tammy, Randy&Kim, Gary&Michelle, Frank, Dominic, Dave, Bob&Pat, Jorge&Cindy, Trish, Brian, Bill, Vivian, Kathy, Tatiana, Cheryl, Stephanie, Howard&Kristine, Len&Colleen, Brian&Rocio, Esther, Drew&Kamila, Sharon, Anne, Sandy, Tony, Dan&Viola, Angie, Susan, Jim, Kelvin, Belinda, Dwayne, Stephen, Kittie, Wendy, Gary&Brenda, Mark&Sandy, Rob&Manya, Karen, Elizabeth, Chris, Pamela, Donna, Rick&Trixie, Jordan, Sheryl, Burton&Wanda.

Disclaimer

I am not a doctor. That should be enough to protect me from those who might take what is in this book and try to create their own treatment regime out of it. But, sadly, it may not be enough. So, let me say it again: I am not a doctor. I talk about a lot of medical procedures and treatments: some of this I got from my own memory, some from doctors, and some from the Internet. Some of it may be wrong. And certainly none of it is in any way related to your medical situation! *I am not a doctor.*

What follows in this book is part anecdote and part advice—general, not medical. None of the anecdotes is intended to be prescriptive, and none of the advice is designed to be your only source of wisdom. Part 3 is presented as conversation with a doctor so as to make it more interesting than a long list of bullet points about cancer, genetics, and prevention. But no real doctor was involved. And even if it were a real conversation with a real doctor, its advice would not be a legitimate alternative to talking to a real doctor. I am but one voice amongst many. Please do not assume that I am the source of more than a modicum of wisdom.

Contents

Part 2: What I Learned from Cancer

Part 3: Conversations with a Doctor

A Final Word

Preface

Tell me, O muse, of that ingenious hero who travelled far and wide after he had sacked the famous town of Troy. Many cities did he visit, and many were the nations with whose manners and customs he was acquainted; moreover he suffered much by sea while trying to save his own life and bring his men safely home; but do what he might he could not save his men, for they perished through their own sheer folly in eating the cattle of the Sun-god Hyperion; so the god prevented them from ever reaching home. Tell me, too, about all these things, O daughter of Jove, from whatsoever source you may know them.

Homer, *The Odyssey*

What follows is a story both substantially and subjectively true. However, it is not consistently objectively true because I did not insist that every chronology was spot-on, nor did I always try to see the narrative from multiple perspectives. This is my personal story, and in it, I tell about my experience of cancer, of doctors, of medicine, and of community.

While I strove at every point to portray my experience fairly, experience itself is far from fair. Thus, I characterize some doctors as heroes and some as villains. That's not to say these were the essential characteristics of these physicians, nor that life breaks down that simplistically, but only that, in my narrative, these persons functioned as heroes and villains to me. A very good friend of mine, who happens also to be a surgeon, said of some of the incidents I have relayed, "That's really hard." When asked to clarify, he responded, "Many of those things you talk about were badly done, yet they are the kinds of things I might have done in the same situation."

All of the things I talk about are true; I did not hyperbolize for the purpose of making the story more interesting. However, in some cases I compressed time, and in other cases, there were minutiae of events or chronology that I felt free to adjust for the sake of the narrative. I expect that, were the doctors in question to recount these same incidents, they might—if they recalled the circumstances at all—offer a different view of some things: we do not remember our unwitting, commonplace activities simply because they may serve as marvellously heroic or spectacularly villainous actions in someone else's narrative.

I have tried to disguise some of the players in this narrative, particularly where the story has the potential to hurt or embarrass. There were other characters for whom I made no such attempt, especially when I wanted to broadcast the depth of gratitude that I have towards them, a gratitude I feel compelled to share publicly. I hope these benefactors will grant me this indulgence and forgive me for making them look so good—yet no better than they truly are.

Introduction

In my opinion, to write a book is for all the world like humming a song—be but in tune with yourself, ... 'tis no matter how high or how low you take it.

Laurence Sterne, *The Life and Opinions of Tristram Shandy, Gentleman*

This is not a story about cancer; it is a story about me. That means you get to listen in on a story which is very personal, but which, at times, will resonate with you. Having told my story to a lot of people, I have often been encouraged to write it down because it is interesting in its own right and because many have wanted to find out what I learned in my journey through cancer. Due to my genetics, this story of mine is ongoing, for even when I do not have an active tumour trying to kill me, I have genes which conspire to allow new ones to develop. Also due to my genetics, my story is a multi-generational tale. One that began, as far back as I have been able to determine from family history, before my maternal grandmother's mother, and continued with my maternal grandmother, then my mother, and finally me. Well, not finally after all, because, as I recently discovered, the story continues with my eldest son. At least this genetic story has a happier component: it is apparent—at least to ourselves—that the genetic woe we have all inherited is happily linked to another trait we have fun sharing—that of genius, with a healthy dose of humour and humility thrown in for good measure!

My writing mentor, Jake MacDonald, said upon hearing me read a portion of this book, "I like it, but it needs to be 5% edgier. Do not hold back for the sake of your potential audience; just tell the story." I considered how to make it edgier, more "real." In the end, though, I realized that was a futile endeavour. When I looked back over the words I'd penned, I didn't see myself holding back so much as just telling my story in my way.

For whatever else it is, this is my story. Finding more edge might make it more interesting to some, but it would ultimately violate my voice—would make it someone else's story, not mine. While the *Fear and Loathing in Winnipeg* version may be rattling around in my head somewhere, that is not the story I am telling today.

So, what I am going to do is to tell my story. A tale, in all its wonderful detail, of me, doctors, hospitals, genetics, crying, laughing, sickness, healing, uncertainty, and overcoming. A tale which drew a bevy of actors into it, from family to friends, from doctors I liked to those I did not. A tale which became a journey in which I was forced to travel along, not like Huck Finn drifting on a raft in the river, subject to all that the river brought, but, instead, like an Olympic kayaker, seeing and anticipating the obstacles and learning to deal deftly with them, albeit sometimes getting very wet.

The book is divided into three sections. While the three parts complement each other and make up one whole, it's important to note that these parts can stand alone and that you can read them in the order you prefer. If you are eager to get your facts straight about cancer, Part 3 will immediately serve you as a kind of primer. If you'd rather hear my seasoned self sharing hard-won lessons with a younger self unaware of the upcoming challenges of cancer, jump straight to Part 2. The book begins with narrative, however, because I believe story is the best place to connect with my readers.

In Part 1, I tell my story in a plain and relatively straightforward manner. I tried not to editorialize too much because I think there is benefit for me in telling the story straight up, and, more importantly, value to you, the reader, in coming to your own conclusions and deducing your own lessons.

Part 2 comprises a series of essays which communicate some of the things I have learned. These are things which I could not put into the narrative without drastically interrupting its flow, but which needed to be said. These are also the things I would have liked to prepare myself with when I was 27 and had cancer for the first time.

Part 3 takes the format of a dialogue with a doctor for the purpose of introducing some of the science of cancer and genetics without sounding like a course lecturer in elementary oncology.

Part 1

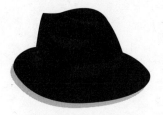

My Story

> *But fortune, good or ill, as I take it,*
> *does not change men and women.*
> *It but develops their characters. As*
> *there are a thousand thoughts lying*
> *within a man that he does not know*
> *till he takes up the pen to write, so the*
> *heart is a secret even to him (or her)*
> *who has it in his own breast.*
>
> William Makepeace Thackeray,
> *The History of Henry Esmond, Esq.*

-1-

In the Beginning

Weary with toil, I haste me to my bed,
The dear repose for limbs with travel tir'd;
But then begins a journey in my head
To work my mind, when body's work's expired.

William Shakespeare, "XXVII" in *Shakespeare's Sonnets*

Somewhere in the dawn of time, matter stirred by the finger of God became life. ... Okay, this story doesn't go back that far, nor is it a tale of mythic proportion. My story does start before I was born, however, for we are each of us the product of our genetics and our environment.

In my case, that reality bears a particular significance. I have an inherited genetic mutation, one of several chromosomal protein deficiencies which together make up a classification called Lynch syndrome. That means I have a gene, reproduced in each cell my body creates, that prevents the proper identification and repair of mutated cells in my body. Unlike the majority of the population, I have a body which allows bad cells to grow and reproduce freely, and eventually this out-of-control reproduction manifests itself as cancer.

Because my story begins with genetics, I look in my family tree to find its start. I look back to my mother, and her mother, and her mother before her. While she was probably not the progenitor of the genetic mutation in my family, my great-grandmother was afflicted with it and is as far back in the family annals as current generations can trace it. The tale stretches not only back through time, however, but also forward. It does not end with me.

The syndrome arises from an autosomal dominant characteristic, meaning that if one parent has it and passes it on, the child will end up with the same condition. It never skips a generation nor are there carriers who do not, in some way, manifest the effects. Because this defective gene, paired with a healthy partner, exists in every chromosomal set in my body, either it or its healthy partner can be passed on at any given time. 50% of the sperm I produce have the defect. Statistically speaking, half of my kids were destined to get this gene, and, right in line with this prediction, one of my three children has the mutation.

As our children approached the age of 18, my wife and I had a conversation with them, and they each, in turn, were tested for the mutated gene. While I love science and math, statistics can be really nasty: when stacked against you, they are, by nature, almost always right. Thus, our middle child (my eldest son) was diagnosed with the syndrome, which means a lifetime of surveillance and testing for him. I'll talk more about these fun father-son events later.

Be as that may, none of this affected my childhood or early adulthood—not until 1992, when I was 27 years old. I had married Debra the previous July and was attending school in a city which was neither my home nor hers: we were creating our own new community of friends. I had a new wife, a new post-graduate degree, and a new prospective career; I had dreams and high hopes for the future. And I was having rectal bleeding.

I was not only bleeding; I was ignoring it. Personal experience had taught me that pain is the primary indicator of a physical problem. If you fall down, twist your leg, and experience pain, you instinctively look at your knee to see what the problem is. Perhaps put ice on it, favour the other leg, or even go to the doctor. But if there is no pain, you feel you can safely ignore the incident. I cannot count the number of soccer and football games I participated in where I finished with blood running down my legs, but there was nothing worse than a cut inflicted, a wound reopened, or just a scrape that would soon scab over. So when I started to experience bleeding but no pain, I more or less ignored it.

"That's a bit strange," I said to myself on more than one occasion. "I thought I had to go to the bathroom, but it was mostly blood. Oh well, it doesn't hurt, and I feel fine, so it will go away."

I am not sure how long this had been happening. When I finally did see a doctor, he asked me that very question.

"How long have you been experiencing these symptoms?"

"I don't know; a few months, maybe."

"Hmmm."

As I ruminated on it later, I expected it could have been a good six months or more that I occasionally bled when I went to the toilet, but with the complete absence of pain and discomfort, I had just let it go. Eventually, though, I'd realized that this was not just going to go away after all, and I'd gone to a walk-in clinic down the road from my house.

I clearly remember the journey. The wind in my face, the sun on my head, the sound of traffic. And I was walking, walking to find out what was wrong, wrong with me.

And with those footsteps, the journey of a thousand miles began. It was April 1992.

The doctor was matter-of-fact in his instructions.

"Let's just check to see if this really is blood. Here is a kit to detect occult blood—meaning it's hidden. When you go to the bathroom, use the enclosed stick to put a sample into the jar. Then bring it back, and we'll have it tested."

I went home and had a chat with my wife, Debra.

"I've been having a bit of bleeding when I go to the bathroom, so I saw the doctor."

Taken aback, her questions tumbled out. "For how long? Are you okay? What did the doctor say?"

"Don't worry; I'm fine. He's just going to do some tests to see what it might be. Nothing hurts, so how bad can it be?"

Debra sounded dubious. "Okaaay." She relented, "Well, let me know what they find."

"Don't worry; I am fine."

The clarion call of the over-confident man. Often a death knell, much like, "Hand me that lighter: I need to see if the gas tank really is empty." We had been married for only 10 months, and Debra did not yet know me as well as she would. History shows that she would not let me get away with that casual approach again.

-2-

Diagnostics

*I saw the cloud, though I did not foresee the storm. It was easy, I say, to see
that their carriage to me was altered, and that it grew worse and worse
every day … .*

Daniel Defoe, *The Fortunes & Misfortunes
of the Famous Moll Flanders &c.*

The next day, faecal sample in hand (in a jar, actually), I headed back to
the clinic to drop off my package. They assured me they'd contact me in
a week or so to let me know what they found. True to their word, about
a week later, I got a call from the clinic to tell me I should go down to
talk with the doctor. When I arrived, I was ushered into the examining
room; the doctor arrived soon after.

"Sir, they found blood in your stool. I will have to schedule you for
another test. You will go to the hospital, and they will do an upper and
lower ultrasound to see if they can find anything wrong."

"Okay."

The doctor gave me an appointment slip for the following week.

That next week I appeared at the hospital for an ultrasound.
It seemed that all the technician could confirm was that I was not
pregnant; she could see nothing wrong.

A couple of days later, I got another call from the clinic. I was to go
see the doctor again to talk about the next step.

"The ultrasound was inconclusive, so we will do a barium enema
next. If this were a bone, we could simply X-ray it, but organs are too
soft to produce the proper contrast for an X-ray. They will have to
introduce barium into your bowel first. Then they will do the X-ray."

"Umm, okay." It sounded like a dubious prospect.

The doctor gave me another appointment slip, once again for the
following week, so off I went.

Now, at this point, you might ask (as I do now but did not have
the insight to do at the time), "Why did they not just send you for a

CT scan? After all, this was 1992, not 1922." Good question—one that I don't have a good answer to. While CT technology was available (confirmed later by its use when I got my second opinion), I am not sure how prevalent it was in the city I was living in, nor am I sure how accessible it was. I know there was not likely to have been more than one in the city, and it may have been that, as a result of the scarcity of this resource, its use was not yet on the list of standard tests to do. Moreover, the doctor wasn't looking for cancer, since I was only 27, and people of that age supposedly don't get cancers of the digestive tract.

Another question you might ask is, "Why is this process taking so long?" Canadians in the crowd will know why. For the others, let me illuminate you: it is the nature of socialized medicine. The byword of the public health vantage point is don't panic; go slow and steady. Cure the disease, but don't do more than you need to; we have to keep costs down. So, rather than scheduling five tests at once, they schedule them sequentially, lest they incur the cost of any tests that might have been unnecessary after a prior test revealed what needed to be known.

In 1991, William Hurt was in a movie called *The Doctor*. In it, he plays a doctor, full of himself and his abilities, who gets cancer and sees the medical system from the inside out. The experience changes his perspective and his life. I think every doctor who deals with gastrointestinal patients should experience two things: a barium enema and a colonoscopy.

If you have not experienced the barium enema, you really ought to get one just to say you have. Essentially, it *is* how it *sounds*—that is, if it sounds to you like something you *wouldn't* want to have done to you! They lay you on your side, stick a tube into your rectum, and then unload a bag of white mush into your large intestine. Barium is a metal that shows up really well on X-rays, so if you coat something with it, it can make a soft organ like your large intestine, or colon, show up really well on an X-ray (think of it as spraying paint onto the Invisible Man). In thinking back over the experience, the procedure was a bit fuzzy in my memory, so I looked it up on the Internet. However, the process described there was nothing like I remembered. The Internet tells me that not only did I use laxatives to purge the contents of my bowels before the procedure, but that the whole procedure was "gentle." That is not my memory. In my memory, there was no preparation for the procedure. Instead, I arrived, they filled me with this stuff, and then I had to stand in this machine while they contorted me about and took X-rays of me in various positions. Then white stuff came out of me for the next couple of days.

Now, cue the doctor's office with yet another appointment.

"The X-rays showed a mass on your large intestine. I have scheduled an appointment with a specialist."

"A mass? What does that mean?"

"Well, it could mean many things. Here is an appointment date and time."

"I understand that it could mean many things. Please tell me some of the things that it could be."

(The doctor was becoming increasingly uncomfortable with my line of questioning.) "Sir, it could be many things. What we know is that there is something on your large intestine. The specialist will be able to give you a better idea."

(Becoming a bit more testy myself.) "I understand. Please tell me some of the things that this could be. Are we talking about a tumour? Cancer?"

"Yes, sir, it could be those things, but let us not jump to conclusions. Instead, go to the specialist, and he will give you a definitive diagnosis."

I left his office with more than a bit of concern in addition to the perpetual appointment slip. As it turned out, it was the last time I would see that doctor: bigger and better things were ahead.

I have never liked to tell people I am worried. My general philosophy is that worrying people before you know what is going on is not very profitable. So when I talked to Debra that day, I tried to be as upbeat as possible. But, in the end, we were both worried and had no answers as to what was happening to me or what this "mass" could be.

The next week, I was off to the specialist.

-3-

Darkness Approaching

O thievish Night,
Why shouldst thou, but for some felonious end,
In thy dark lantern thus close up the stars
That Nature hung in heaven, and filled their lamps
With everlasting oil, to give due light
To the misled and lonely traveller?

John Milton, *Comus*

I wish doctors were more creative in designing their waiting rooms. I figure there is some course in generic design offered in medical school to ensure that all waiting rooms are box-shaped, with identical chairs set up in the same configurations. And they all have subscriptions to the same magazines. How do they consistently get the same vintage issues? Perhaps the special supplier where doctors buy these things? One where a kindly clerk greets you and asks, "Looking for the May 1978 edition of *Canadian Home Gardening*? Why, yes, here it is."

Waiting in the specialist's office, I overheard conversations with statements such as, "I am so grateful to Dr. X; he saved my life!" Word of mouth advertising is always the best. I felt better already.

I stepped into his office, where he sat across from me, a big desk in between us.

"So, how the hell did you get this?"

"Not sure. It's not even clear to me what I have."

"They found a four-centimetre mass on your rectum. Here is what we are going to do." (I love how doctors tend to say "we" when what they really mean is "what I will do to you.")

"I will insert a rigid scope into you and take a look inside. If I can visualize the mass, I'll cut off a piece and send that to the lab, so we can figure out what it is. If it comes back as benign, then I can go back in, and we'll gouge it out. If it is more serious, then we can determine a course of action at that time."

"So, it could be cancer?"

"Let's worry about that later."

Feeling reassured and a bit more educated, I went into his examining room, and he conducted his exam as promised. The exam was not very pleasant, as it consisted of him pushing a long rigid tube into my rectum and then clipping a piece off of the intestinal wall, but it was tolerable and short-lived.

As I left the examining room, I was still a bit worried but confident that I was in good hands.

A few days later, I got a call from this latest specialist.

"Please come down to the hospital to meet me, and bring your wife. I will be waiting."

As I hung up the phone, I was no longer confident. Something was wrong; if not, he would neither have insisted that I meet him right away nor asked me to bring Debra along. She and I did not talk as we rode our bikes to the hospital, only a couple of blocks from our apartment.

When we arrived at the hospital, we were ushered into a large conference room with a huge boardroom table in it. We sat on one side, and when the doctor entered the room, he sat close to the door, seemingly as far away from us as he could.

"You have cancer, and I have scheduled you for surgery next week. Given the position and size of the tumour, its removal will necessitate that I close off your anus and create a colostomy, an opening in your side where we will have to attach a bag to collect your waste. In addition, it is very likely that the surgery will render you impotent. Now, you can get other opinions, but I have consulted with 10 doctors at CancerCare here in town, and this is the recommended treatment. A couple of my patients have gone to California for less radical surgeries to avoid the colostomy, but things did not turn out well, and they returned to me for the original treatment. My office will contact you with the instructions for the surgery. You can stay in this room as long as you need to. Here are some tissues, if you need to cry."

He paused briefly, and then, getting up, he left the room. It would be the last I saw of him. It was May 29th, 1992, and it had taken eight weeks to figure out that I had cancer.

-4-

The First of Many Tears

Heaven knows we need never be ashamed of our tears, for they are rain upon the blinding dust of earth, overlying our hard hearts.

Charles Dickens, *Great Expectations*

We cried.

I sat with my wife as my future, my hopes, and my dreams washed away in my tears. We were confused and hurt, and disbelieving despair was beginning to set in as we exited the room and walked out of the hospital into the bright afternoon. Even the sunlight seemed harsh.

As soon as we got home from the hospital, I did two things. First, I wrote the one and only journal entry of my life. In it, I vented my anger and lamented the imminent loss of my manhood and my bowel function. Not yet one year into my marriage, and I was to be rendered impotent, with a bag to collect faeces permanently attached to my side.

Second, and ultimately life-changing, I called Ken Bayly, a doctor and friend in my hometown of Saskatoon.

"Hi, Dr. Bayly. I have no idea what to do and hope you can help me. I just got a cancer diagnosis from a specialist, and here is what he says he wants to do."

I explained what the specialist had told me.

"Exactly where is the cancer—how high up? And what stage is it?"

"Other than being in my rectum somewhere, I have no idea. And he didn't say anything about the stage either."

"Well, it's odd that he's so definitive about his treatment and its results, but he didn't tell you the placement of the tumour or how advanced it is. If I were in your place, I'd want a second opinion. Tell you what: I have a friend who is a surgeon. I can get you in to see him on Monday, and he'll give you a second opinion."

With a large measure of relief for this support, and feeling as though I were getting the best medical care, I gratefully agreed to be there first thing Monday morning. It was late in the afternoon on Friday, I cried again as I thanked Dr. Bayly and hung up the phone. You'll notice that I cry a lot.

I called my friend Don, who had been best man at my wedding and was living in Japan at the time.

"*Konnichiwa*. ... Hello."

"I have cancer."

We talked, and I cried. And the thing I remember most prominently after he prayed for me was that he said, "I feel so far away."

"I feel so far away." I have felt the same when experiencing from a distance the tragedies of people whom I love. Far away can be physical distance, but it can also be time and psychological separation. It can be the revelation that, years earlier, someone you were close to experienced the break-up of his marriage. It is the knowledge that your brother has experienced a mental breakdown, and there is little you can do. It is hearing about the terminal illness of someone who is physically far away. It is the realization that there is no substitute for a touch or the ability to look into someone's eyes, feel his pain, and give him comfort.

The rest of the weekend was a blur. We made preparations for the trip home, just a two-and-a-half hour drive. I called my family: my dad in Saskatoon first, telling him I was coming up and why. I called my mom, living in Winnipeg, to tell her the shocking news. And I called Saskatoon again, to let a close friend know I would be in town. Debra, who was a sessional lecturer at the University of Regina at the time, called her boss to make preparations to be away for a couple of days. And she called her family and friends.

Even at that time, I felt my community begin to be conspicuously present to me. Debra and I went out that evening to visit friends, sharing supper and a movie and ruminating over the presence of God and his role in our suffering. Saturday morning our pastor came over to pray for me. Sunday I called together the leadership of our church, some of whom I'd developed a rather strained relationship with, and asked them to pray for me. I would comment later that, despite the failings of the church both in general and in my own life, there were times when it approached the caring community that it was meant to be. This proved to be one of those times.

There are many stories built into the silent spaces of my own story, stories about what others went through during my journey. It's easy for me to forget or gloss over their experiences: my wife tells me that I can lack empathy at times. Not only is it hard for me to read people, but

I also have a hard time reading circumstances. This means that I take people at face value when, in fact, there may be deeper currents running.

So, when I'd called my parents to tell them of my diagnosis, I had been matter-of-fact, and, by all appearances, so had they. But looks can be deceiving. I can recall my dad crying in my presence just once in my life, as he'd sat in an empty house and told me my mother had left. On that day, however, after I'd called with my cancer diagnosis, he had cried as he'd spoken to his brother about my illness.

And, while I was busy with my life and my own issues, countless people, many of whom I was not even aware of, held me up with their tears and with their prayers. There would be an ocean of tears cried before my story was done.

-5-

Cancer Changes Everything

Thus, we never see the true state of our condition till it is illustrated to us by its contraries, nor know how to value what we enjoy, but by the want of it.

Daniel Defoe, *The Life and Adventures of Robinson Crusoe*

In the movie *Apollo 13*, there was, for me, a profound and memorable scene. It had nothing to do with the accident nor its resolution. Nor was it the mission control proclamation, "Not on my watch!" It was simply the brief scene in Jim Lovell's back yard when he sat with his wife looking up at the moon after the telecast of the first moon landing. The moon winked in and out of view as he alternately covered and then uncovered it with his thumb. And he said, "Today we live in a world where man has walked on the moon."

The world had not really changed. Technology had not advanced measurably in the moment when Neil Armstrong stepped out onto the surface of the moon, and Armstrong himself was not a fundamentally different person in skills or personality. But, everything had changed in that wondrous moment when we, as a race, realized there was no obstacle we could not overcome if we put our collective will, effort, and pocketbook behind a solution.

My cancer diagnosis did not really change anything, not physically anyway. The pronouncement, "You have cancer," did not make me physically better or worse off than I'd been a moment earlier. My tumour was neither bigger nor smaller than it had been the minute before I learned of its presence. Nonetheless, cancer changed everything. I was a different, radically broken person. I had a new fear about the future that I had been free of the moment before. I had questions about God, about myself, my relationships, stability, and the goodness of the world. And I had questions about who I was, what I was doing, and what I might have done to have caused this awful thing growing inside me. At that moment of revelation, I became someone with cancer.

I also became someone on a mission to change—something, anything—about my life that might make this tumour easier to beat. And in that quest, I reached far beyond what I would have grasped for in my more lucid moments and fastened onto things that, for the most part, I held for only a brief time before quickly abandoning.

I embraced vegetarianism. Overnight I abandoned all meat, thinking that there must be something significant in my diet that had caused this gastrointestinal tumour, and that the something might be meat. The day after my diagnosis, I was choking down eggplant casserole, courtesy of a supportive friend, and barbecuing tofu "wieners." My desperation did not, unfortunately, extend to cooperation from my taste buds, and I did not find the new fare pleasing to my palate. Until then, I had never realized how many billboards focused on food, nor, of those, how many depicted meat! But I started to notice then: they seemed to be everywhere, and I found them quite distracting.

I started running again. I have always had a love–hate relationship with solitary physical activity. A soccer player, I had played team sports regularly until my mid-twenties. But at that point, while I was at school in Regina, opportunities had become harder to find, so my participation had dwindled. I was rapidly becoming the stereotypical couch potato. However, cancer gave me a renewed incentive to get back into shape, so I started running on a daily basis.

I became committed to homeopathy, the alternative medicine based on the principle of inoculation. Trace amounts of substances which would normally produce the symptoms you have instead create an immuno-counterresponse, resulting in the body healing itself naturally. I must admit that, having met a friend only a couple of years earlier who was a practicing homeopath, I, along with others in our group of mutual friends, had done my share of scoffing at this treatment strategy. However, cancer changed that. After all, what harm could it do? And if it worked, even a bit, would it not be worthwhile? In fact, Debra and I became so enamoured with this idea that we would make a 16-hour round trip from Regina to Edmonton to get an evaluation and enough pills to take me through the waiting period until my surgery. (Of course, the fact that it was dear friends who practiced the homeopathy added great incentive to visit them.)

Looking back, I can see that the radical changes I made to my life in the wake of my cancer diagnosis were not harmful, but neither were they particularly helpful. In my deep-seated fear of the future, I needed to do something, anything, to try to take back control of my life and my health. And for that reason, what I did was good. But the reality is that none of these things stuck. I went a mere 30 days before I embraced my inner carnivore again. I think that the running had already disappeared shortly before that, and the homeopathy was discontinued once I ran out of my initial prescription.

Good lifestyle is important in the prevention of and recovery from cancer: I cannot stress that enough. But individual actions are not lifestyle, and the changes in my actions were not changes in my lifestyle. They were, simply put, panic. They were my challenge to the spectre of uncertainty that cancer presented to me. And that challenge, while psychologically useful for a time, did not create any lasting change.

-6-

Second Opinion

It is a narrow mind which cannot look at a subject from various points of view.

George Eliot, *Middlemarch*

My wife and I are two different kinds of shoppers. Frankly, I hate shopping and will do whatever I can to get in and out of a store as quickly as possible. In fact, there was one year I abandoned Christmas presents entirely because I got into the mall and was so overwhelmed by the mayhem and crush of the crowds that I just went home, perhaps having encountered a latent phobia of some kind. When I go to shop, I enter the store with a fixed idea of what I want, where it is, and the path to and from the item. My wife is just the opposite; she loves to shop. She loves the idea of comparing between one store and another and between one item and another. I even joked with her when we were shopping for our current house that, had she been able, she would have bought three homes, lived in each one for a while, and then returned the two she did not want. I, on the other hand, do not like choice, and, for the most part, I just want an expert to tell me which item or course of action is best, and then I'll move forward with that. It's not that I'm incapable of weighing options or don't think that it's useful to do so, but, in unimportant or less critical things, I'd just like my life to be simple. Sometimes I long for the days of Henry Ford, when I could get any colour car, as long as it was black.

I've discovered that this need to have an expert tell me what to do is very prevalent in the general population regarding matters of medicine. We go to the doctor with an ache or a pain and put ourselves into her hands. Often, and without thinking, we open our mouth, say "Awwww," and then swallow the pill she prescribes. What is it about doctors that makes us trust so unquestioningly?

I once heard Margaret Somerville, an ethicist and the head of the Centre for Medicine, Ethics, and Law at McGill University in Montreal, speak about our view of authority figures in general and of doctors in particular. To paraphrase her comments, there was a time when we exercised blind faith in doctors and fully accepted the premise that they should be believed in all things medical because of their title. Now, however, we require earned trust; we demand that they prove their expertise to us over time.

I have been both witness and party to this paradigm shift. As a baby boomer, I was taught that it is right to trust those in authority. Many so-called millennials, on the other hand, seem to be born with an inherent mistrust of authority figures. I grew up subscribing to blind faith in doctors. In the course of my journey through cancer, however, I learned how to mistrust medical professionals, and my faith is no longer blind.

On Monday morning, June 1st, Debra and I arrived in the hospital at the appointed time. I was taken to an examining room, and in came the surgeon, Dr. Joseph Pfeifer. He greeted me warmly but with earnest respect for the gravity of the situation. He then sat down with the whiteboard he'd brought in and drew a picture of my digestive system.

"Okay, here is your large intestine," he began, pointing to the diagram he'd just drawn, "and here is roughly where the tumour is. Its exact placement will help determine which surgical procedure I use," he continued. "I'm going to do a manual exam now to find out if I can feel it, and then I'm going to send you for a CT scan to see if we can get a good picture of what we are dealing with."

He pulled out the rubber gloves and, with the typical snap, put them on. With lube sufficient to cover his whole hand, he conducted his exam.

"Well, I can't feel anything there. That means the tumour is more than a few centimetres up into your rectum. That's a good sign because it means it may be possible to surgically remove it without having to resort to a colostomy. Those kinds of things are only done if there's not sufficient tissue left at the anus end of the colon to reconnect the two ends after resection, or removal, of the portion with the tumour. So, off to the CT room, and I'll see you in a couple of hours."

Hooray! A new test. I left Debra sitting in the hallway, whence she was to watch me for the next couple of hours, begowned and beslippered in the nicest hue of hospital blue, scuttling back and forth and in and out of various doors. (She said it reminded her of *Noises Off,* for any of you familiar with the classic comedy about the goings-on behind the scenes as a stage play is supposedly being performed.)

First, there was prep for the CT scan. I had to drink a great quantity of liquid and then wait for it to inflate my bladder to ensure we got a good picture. The process was challenging: I was sure I was going to explode or just wet myself as I lay on the table being run in and out of the scanner. Once that test was done, and I was able to visit the facilities, I met with Dr. Pfeifer again.

"Looks like a mass, for sure. I've booked a room so we can do a sigmoidoscopy. That's a scope with a light and a camera at the end. We'll use an enema to clean out your rectum first, and then I'll insert the scope into you. That will let me get a good look at the tumour and also get a biopsy of it."

More prep and then the scope.

One of my favourite TV shows was *The Operation,* where the real-life surgery that was shown fascinated me. I've long wished I could have my own procedures filmed, especially the surgeries, for my later viewing pleasure. However, this would perhaps be too gruesome as well as too telling of what actually goes on in an operating room, what with all the machines that go "ping" and everyone looking around to account for that one clamp that seems to be missing but no one can quite put their finger on.

Suffice it to say, I love science. And I have always particularly loved medical science, so the prospect of being able to see my insides was thrilling. As Dr. Pfeifer was conducting the scope, there was a monitor on which I could watch his progress, ask endless questions, and see first-hand this tumour that I had. He got to the site and took several pictures; a pincer then came out of the end of his instrument and grabbed my intestinal wall. Pulling a bit, it tore off a piece of tissue which then got sucked out of me. The sensation was odd, since I could feel the pull and, on the monitor, see the blood, yet I felt no pain.

This, I found out, is the limitation of the nerves in the intestine and underscored one of the bad assumptions I'd made. It seems that your intestine has nerves sensitive only to expansion, such as you feel when you have pain from gas. However, your intestine does not have nerves to detect the pain of cutting. So when I experienced bleeding but no pain, it was not a reliable indicator that everything was fine because my intestine simply had no capacity to detect the kind of malady I had. In fact, if pain does accompany your bleeding, you are probably in better shape than if you have bleeding without pain.

Once the procedure was complete, Dr. Pfeifer left to see if he could get a rush on the pathology. About an hour passed, I estimate, and he came back.

"Well, if you had not known already, I would have some bad news for you—you have cancer."

I nodded.

"This is what I can tell you. The tumour is far enough up into your rectum—about 10 centimetres—that I think I can take it out and safely reattach everything. This will leave you pretty much intact, the same as you are now. In addition, the idea that you will be impotent is improbable. I don't know why it was ever mentioned. First, impotence is very much in your head. Second, I would have to be pretty sloppy to do enough nerve damage to guarantee impotence. I will try to do a better job than that."

Night and day.

Up until this point, I had done a lot of waiting. Every time there was a new test, a new procedure, I'd had to wait, first to get the procedure and then to get the results. Now that I had a firm diagnosis and a much improved prognosis, the longest wait of all was to begin. Knowing I had cancer, and not having any frame of reference with which to be able to judge the severity or rapidity with which it was growing, I would wait, keenly aware that this menacing threat continued to increase its territory inside me.

With this knowledge of what was wrong, but with the assurance from Dr. Pfeifer that he would book an operating theatre on an urgent basis (within two to four weeks), Debra and I went home with much lighter hearts than we had arrived. When we got back, I called the first surgeon, and, with a certain amount of smugness but a greater sense of relief, told his receptionist that I would not be requiring his services.

The Waiting

Time flies over us, but leaves its shadow behind.

Nathaniel Hawthorne, *The Marble Faun*

Tom Petty is not the only one to notice that waiting is the hardest thing; he just wrote the best music to that inner monologue. I have found that the difficulty has less to do with the actual amount of time that passes and more to do with the uncertainty that builds in its space. There is a considerable difference between being in an uncomfortable (or terrifying) situation and knowing it will end than having to wait with no knowledge of when, or even if, the pain or distress will be over.

While in retrospect I know that the tumour I had was still in its relative infancy and that I was in no danger of its growth overwhelming me in the four weeks I awaited word of a space in the hospital, at that time I had no such assurance. So, each day Debra and I anxiously awaited the call to "come on down." And each day we were disappointed and became that much more anxious about what was to become of me. It felt as though I had a device planted inside me that would suddenly, without warning, explode, perhaps killing me in my sleep.

In the middle of this protracted wait, I had a visitor whose arrival was designed to allay my fears about the worst-case scenario. While Dr. Pfeifer had assured me he was going to put me back together as close to original specifications as he could, there was still an outside chance that a colostomy would be required. If that were the case, rather than resecting, or removing, a piece of my large intestine and then attaching the two free ends back together to create an anastomosis, a more complicated resolution would be required. First, the part of the rectum which was closest to the anus would have to be permanently closed off, essentially sewing the anus shut. Second, a hole, or stoma, would be cut into my abdomen, and the other end of the rectum would then be sewn onto the stoma. This would have the effect of routing my waste through my waist. Left simply like that, however, this arrangement would be utterly impractical, smelly, and messy, so a connection point would be created at the stoma to allow a colostomy bag to be fastened to it. Thus, whenever faeces exited my body—no longer a voluntarily controlled process—the mess would end up in the bag, which I would then clean out at my convenience.

Transition to being a patient with a stoma is not without its psychological trauma, both before and after the procedure. So, when patients are facing the possibility of such a procedure, the local Ostomy Association finds a volunteer who is similar in age and lifestyle to you, and you meet to talk. The guy who came to my house was nice enough and appeared to be about my age. His case differed from mine as he had had ulcerative colitis, a debilitating disease of the bowel which is replete with pain, intestinal distress, and bleeding ulcers. After years of torment, he had finally had his entire large intestine removed, leaving him with an ileostomy—a connection between his small intestine and a bag attached to his side.

"Things are not so bad with a stoma. I have a girlfriend, and we just went skiing. The bag cramps my lifestyle a bit, but not nearly as much as the pain from my colitis did. Best thing that ever happened to me."

"What about diet?"

"I have to take a little care in what I eat. While my mouth does not know the difference, my GI process does: it's kind of embarrassing when I drink too much beer or Coke, and the bag fills up with gas."

When he'd left, I found myself musing that the visit had not really accomplished what it was designed to do. While I am thankful for people like this volunteer because many people would indeed find great comfort in his assurance that life goes on after radical surgery, the meeting had not resonated well with me. In the end, all his visit had done was to reinforce in my mind the potentiality of an outcome I'd been told was possible but not very likely. Thus, an evening that had started out with pleasant conversation suddenly left me shaken, if only for the next few hours, to realize how serious and possibly life-changing my situation really was, regardless of the reassurances I'd received from the doctor I was now relying on for my health and wholeness.

After having waited for about four weeks, I called my friend Dr. Bayly on a Friday to find out whether he could tell me anything.

"Doc, I am worried. How much longer is it going to be?"

"It has been too long. Look, here is what we're going to do. Prepare to come out this weekend. I'll push to get an operating theatre for you on Monday, but if I can't arrange that, we'll just check you in through emergency and say your bleeding has increased and you need surgery right away."

That seemed to me a somewhat dodgy approach, but I was feeling as though I really needed to do something. As we prepared to leave for Saskatoon though, I got a call I'd been waiting for: the hospital had a space was ready for me. I would be checking into the hospital on Sunday morning.

-8-

The First Surgery

Let us go then, you and I,
When the evening is spread out against the sky
Like a patient etherized upon a table ...

T.S. Eliot, *The Love Song of J. Alfred Prufrock*

Surgical procedures have been around since the dawn of time. In Neolithic times, trephination, the practice of drilling holes through the skull, was popular and widespread, perhaps perceived as a way to release evil spirits. It had the added advantage of actually helping reduce damage from swelling caused by blows to the head, provided that the patient survived the procedure and accompanying infection. Amputations have been common and necessary throughout the history of civilizations rife with both accident and war. And, astoundingly, invasive surgeries were common even before the invention of anaesthetic in the 1840s, thanks to strong men and leather straps to hold down the patient and alcoholic beverages to dull the pain. Even after the advent of anaesthetic, the lack of knowledge about bacteria and the need for cleanliness meant that many people still died as a result of post-operative complications, although more patients were surviving the surgery itself. Today, surgery has advanced far beyond its ancient days: many of its risks now arise from the complexity of modern procedures are and our attempt to repair bodies that are more and more damaged.

I arrived at the hospital in Saskatoon on Sunday, June 28th, with a surgery scheduled for the next day, exactly four weeks from the day I'd received my diagnosis and surgical plan from Dr. Pfeifer. I was installed in a *quad,* designed to hold up to four individuals. Two other guys were in my room when I arrived, but by the time I eventually went home, I was alone. One guy was an elderly gentleman, Mr. Penner, a kindly old man. I'm not sure why he was there, but he was gone by Tuesday. The second guy was a younger man, probably in his mid-30s. As I arrived, I noticed his wife, who looked familiar to me. After I'd been in the room a few minutes, I recognized them both as a couple from my church in Saskatoon. It seems he'd experienced a bowel obstruction as the result of a prior procedure and had just gone through the same surgery I was about to have, albeit having been admitted as an emergency patient. He was two days ahead of me, so it was an encouragement over the next week and a half to see what my recovery would look like two days hence.

There was a lot of preparation to get ready for my surgery. Of course, I had to don the standard backless gown typical of the hospitality of the medical system. Then there were pills to take ("This one kills the bacteria in your intestinal tract—the good ones will come back eventually"), shots to get, visits from doctors ("This is Dr. Jones; he will be your anaesthesiologist"), and, finally, a disturbing visit from an ostomy nurse.

A friend of mine once broke his femur (the large bone at the top of the leg) in a skiing accident. As part of the treatment, he had a metal rod, as well as various other pieces of metal hardware, temporarily implanted in his leg. When it came time to remove them again, he found himself in the hospital. During the pre-operative procedure, his surgeon entered the room, examined his legs, and then, taking out a permanent black marker, wrote on his good leg, "NOT THIS ONE." Now that's just good planning.

For me, there was no writing, but there was a bit of colouring, being sure to stay inside the lines. The nurse, having pulled out a black marker, said, "Even though Dr. Pfeifer does not anticipate he will have to give you a colostomy, we have to measure and mark you anyway. An ostomy would be permanent, so we have to ensure that any hole he needs to cut in your side when you're under anaesthetic is in the right place."

"Okay," I assented reluctantly. This worried me more than a little.

The nurse had me stand up and adjust my hospital pants to a comfortable position. Then she drew a large circle on the left side of my abdomen just above the waistline with her marker. That was disconcerting, to say the least.

Evening came, and I got the first of two pre-surgery enemas to clean me out as well as they could. Then it was just a waiting game.

Later on, Dr. Pfeifer came by to talk briefly with me about what to expect the next morning: to tell me how the surgery was going to go and to reassure me that things would be alright. I knew he was a Christian guy, so, before he left, I asked him to pray with Debra and me. We prayed that God would guide his hands and his mind as he performed the surgery the next day. It was profoundly reassuring.

Then the wait, again.

The next morning, I was up bright and early. A final enema to complete the cleansing, a kiss for my wife who had braided my long hair to keep it out of the way during the operation, and I was off, like a shot.

I love the orderlies who frequent the hallways of hospitals. But there must be a certain kind of crazy training they all have to go through or a test they have to pass before they can get hired. I am sure the orderly who wheeled my bed from my room to the operating theatre got his lessons from some odd Mario-Andretti-meets-demolition-derby hybrid, because we careened through the halls of the hospital, bouncing off walls and calling out as we came around blind corners, laughing and talking the whole time. His style was that of a cab driver I'd had in Trinidad once, slowing at blind intersections, honking twice to let people know he was there, and then barrelling through with no consideration for his passenger sitting tensely with hands clenched and blanched face.

When we finally got to the operating theatre, the orderly parked me outside the door and knocked. Out came a bemasked surgeon, who quickly pronounced, "This is not my patient." I looked up to see a female surgeon: she was definitely not my doctor. Glad I would not be having someone attempt to perform a hysterectomy on me before realizing I was a man, I asked my orderly to move us on quickly! Thankfully, there was Dr. Pfeifer to greet me.

"Good-morning, Dennis. Good to see you."

I smiled weakly.

I was wheeled into the theatre and transferred onto the operating table, then asked to sit up. I remember the words of the anaesthesiologist at that point.

"I am going to poke you a bit here in the back to freeze you, and then I am going to put a line in here. Little poke. Good. Now, I am just going to insert the line. That doesn't hurt, does it? Okay, now, I'll just give you a bit of anaesthetic to relax you. If you could just count down from ... ."

I did not even get to start the count.

-9-

Hospital Recovery

So,—now, the danger dared at last,
Look back, and smile on perils past!

Sir Walter Scott, *The Bridal of Triermain*

General anaesthetic, necessary for major surgery, is not like sleeping. There is no fitful wakefulness; there are no dreams. There is awake, and then there is not awake, followed by sudden awake again, with the accompanying sense that no time has passed but with a heavy grogginess that comes from having been unconscious for an undetermined amount of time.

Time had passed. And with that passing time, things had happened. A squadron of medical people kept me alive while a man with a knife first did extensive damage to me and then managed to repair that damage. In another location in the same hospital, people fussed and talked and laughed together. Some of them hugged and cried and prayed. They told stories and remembered fun and life, but, as if to avoid both the discomfort and risk of certain topics, there was no discussion of death or colostomies. In locations outside of the hospital, beyond the city and even the country, still others worried, but many alone and in silence, some praying to God to guide the surgeon's hands and to spare my life for the good that was to come in it.

Many of those things, both profound and ordinary, happened without prompting and without fanfare. I discovered only recently, in the course of writing this book, that during my surgery and hospitalization, my mother-in-law, vacationing in Europe, had prayed in every cathedral she and my father-in-law had visited, offering up prayers for my safety and healing. I also know that many people whom I barely knew but who were friends of my wife and her family had gathered together for mutual support and to pray that God's will would be done in my life.

The relief was far more profound to these faithful people than it was to me, still "under," when the surgeon finally appeared with the news that, despite significant struggle and some complications, the surgery had been successful and everything was going to be alright. Debra left the hospital for the first time that day, enjoying a walk in the bright sun with a spring in her step and a broad smile on her face, feeling for all the world that, with present danger passed, nothing in our world could ever be wrong again. For me, lying in the recovery room, the light was just dimly beginning to go on again.

I remember waking up in the recovery room with a nurse looking over me. My first response to this sudden consciousness was to move my hand down to my side, to the black mark the ostomy nurse had painted on me, to see what permanent changes had been made: nothing. What a relief! That arduous task out of the way, I lapsed back into unconsciousness, and the next thing I knew I was back in my room.

The surgery itself had not proceeded as smoothly as hoped, going over-length by a full two hours—each minute of which had caused Debra growing anxiety. My understanding is that opening me up and resecting the tumour had been pretty straightforward. However, once the task came to join the two parts back together, problems had begun. Between my narrow male hips and the low placement of the tumour, access to the short length of tissue on the anal end was severely impeded. Dr. Pfeifer's surgical team brilliantly completed the anastomosis, however.

A nifty surgical device which had only recently come into use ended up saving the day. In the deft hands of Dr. Pfeifer and the partner he'd called in to assist when the going got really tough, this tool facilitated what would otherwise have been impossible. The implement they used consists of one piece inserted into the anus and another piece fitted over the tissue on the other end to be attached. Then, swish, it brings the two pieces of tissues together, one inside the other, and staples them, trimming the excess tissue. Another important piece of surgical equipment had been the table itself, which Dr. Pfeifer had tilted and swung around at every possible angle for optimum access to the anastomosis site. Like da Vinci's Vitruvian man on a surgical tilt-a-whirl, I had hung right side up and upside down on various planes of inclination throughout the day.

Altogether, the team had been presented with an almost overwhelming challenge to put me together. Dr. Pfeifer reported to my wife that he had fought for well over two hours trying to reattach the plumbing, as it were; it is a tribute to both his determination and skill that I did not end up with a colostomy. He said that in the back of his mind had been two thoughts: first, that I was still a young man, too young to be permanently altered if at all avoidable; and two, that any changes he made were going to be permanent, so he had better bring to bear every skill and all the perseverance he had. With that battle won, he had finally closed me up, and the operation was complete.

The first day of my recovery was kind of a blur. What I do remember is tubes, and a lot of them. In addition to 25 staples to hold me together, I woke up with a central line in my neck (an intravenous line that ran into the jugular vein in my neck and down into my vena cava, just above the heart), an epidural in my lower back (for pain control), a nasogastric (NG) tube (a tube in my nose that went down into my stomach to drain the fluids until my digestive system started working again), a catheter (enough said about that), and an abdominal drain (a ball hanging at the end of a tube that was inserted into my side to drain waste fluid from the incision site inside me). Over the course of the next week and a half, the tubes all came out, one at a time. Each time, the nurse would say something like this:

"Okay, this is going to come out. It's going to hurt a bit, but it will be over quickly."

And then some tube would get removed. Some were quick and easy—hmmm, no, I take that back. They were all far more involved than I expected, and each one left me thinking, "*That* was in me?" The best one, and I use the word "best" in terms of memorability only, was the drain. The abdominal drain, which could not be removed until it had stopped collecting waste fluid from inside at the anastomosis site, was the last tube to come out, nine days after surgery.

Keep in mind that the moment your body receives a trauma, it goes into repair mode, trying the best it can to fix the damage done. So when a surgeon pokes a hole into your side and inserts a tube, your body has a significant desire to repair that hole. It is only the presence of the tube that keeps the hole from healing over completely. Also keep in mind that healing happens as deeply inside the body as the trauma occurs. Thus, in addition to trying to heal the surface wounds, my body was trying to heal its deep tissue as well.

Now, the drain is an interesting device, essentially a tube going into the abdominal wound with a removable ball at the outer end. This ball can be taken off and emptied; it is then squeezed before being reattached to the tube so as to create a slight suction to draw off excess fluid that has developed in the body cavity. Fifteen years down the road, after my second surgery, I would reflect on the fact that I'd had this device only during my first surgery. Initially, I thought the device must be unique to Saskatchewan, as unique as the term *bunny hug* to denote a pull-over sweatshirt with a hood. However, I recently learned that the device has simply been archived because it's not particularly effective in speeding healing. Despite this fact, I steadfastly maintain that it was some kind of punishment for an unknown peccadillo of mine, although I cannot think what might have been of sufficient magnitude to warrant such torment.

In order to keep the drain tube from slipping out of me when I moved around, its inner length culminated in a flared end, like a rubber arrow. I can imagine that the drain is inserted when the patient's abdomen is open, the wound then sutured up, and the drain tube pulled out until the flared end comes up against the abdominal wall. Regardless of the methodology employed, the head is larger than the tube, and, consequently, larger than the hole through which the tube passes. Now consider the length of time elapsed since my surgery, as well as the desire of my body to heal itself by closing this hole, and perhaps an image of the proverbial square peg in a round hole springs to your mind as it does to mine.

Here is the way the extraction went. The part of the patient is played by me, the other by one of my kindly nurses.

"Okay, Dennis, this is really going to hurt a lot."

"Uh-huh."

"Now, it is very important that when I begin to pull, you stay relaxed because, if you tense up your abdominal muscles, it will be harder to get the tube out."

"Uh-huh."

"Here we go."

At this point, she began to pull the tube out.

Think about the last time you had a trauma to the abdomen. If you are a boxer or had regular fights on the playground as a kid, you will know how your body responds to being punched in the abdomen. In the event you are not familiar with this, let me describe it for you. When your abdomen receives a blow, your body instinctively prepares for a second blow. This is accomplished by—wait for it—tightening up the muscles. That way, if another blow arrives, it will be met with an appropriately hardened abdominal wall ready to withstand the blow, serving to protect the internal organs.

"Ahhhhhhh!" (That is a cry of pain, not me opening my mouth so that she can have a look inside.)

"Relax! Relax! You have to relax!"

"I am trying to relax! Stop doing this to me, and I can relax!"

Finally, the drain was out, and I felt as though I had given birth. Well, not really, but at that point I had no frame of reference for such an experience; it was certainly the most pain I'd felt to date. I must admit I found an entirely new register for my pain scale many years later when I tried to walk down the stairs after my first Ironman, but that is a different book.

But I've jumped too far ahead; let me go back a couple of tubes. It was a grand day of rejoicing when the NG tube was removed, because not only did it get the irritation out of my throat, but it meant that I could begin the slow progression towards being able to eat.

The rest of my hospital stay amounted to a series of anecdotes. No complications, no issues, just waiting for my intestines to "wake up" and for my drain to stop producing fluid. Dr. Pfeifer had removed about 15 centimetres of my rectum, and pathological testing of the tumour and of the surrounding tissue that was removed had categorized the tumour as stage IA. This notation signified that the tumour had been fully contained within the intestinal wall and had no lymph node involvement. As a result, no cancer-related follow-up was required: no radiation, no chemotherapy.

Ten days in the hospital is like a year in solitary confinement, or so it can seem to the uninitiated. There is nowhere to go and nothing to do, really. No TV, no Internet (not in those days), and too little well-being to enjoy reading. I am not sure how I survived in such a wasteland. For the first six or seven days, I could not eat because my intestines were still figuring out how to recover from the trauma they had faced. Bowel surgery is an excellent, although somewhat radical, weight-loss regime, I must admit; I lost 25 pounds in that time, as I was to do again later during my second hospitalization 15 years later. In the present case, I dropped from 190 back to my high school weight of 165.

I did get a cool gadget on the first day after surgery: called an incentive spirometer, it was a plastic gizmo with a hollow ball inside and a protruding flexible hose. Imagine the hose as a large bendable straw, with a mouthpiece attached to the end. It seems that after having general anaesthetic, your lungs have a tendency not to work correctly, so you use this device to help them recover. Basically, you suck air from the mouthpiece into your lungs. To ensure that you do it correctly—that is, with sufficient force—you watch the ball on the inside: it rises in the vacuum tube as you draw air. You are doing the exercise correctly if you can get the ball to hover between the two lines near the top for the duration of a slow inhale. It was the closest thing to a video game that I had available to me and provided many minutes of breathtaking entertainment.

The pain from my surgery was tolerable, except for the gnawing in my stomach from not being able to eat anything more than ice chips. Even then, the nurses admonished, "Don't swallow too much—that's just so you have something to put in your mouth." After the first day, the tubes became irritating, especially the NG tube, which was bothering my throat when I swallowed. Nonetheless, despite having manual control over the epimorph line running into my back, I stopped taking pain killers after the second day because I disliked the effect of light-headedness; I preferred the sensation of low-grade pain with a clear head to feeling "out of it" all the time.

Unlike the very early days of modern medicine, it is now axiomatic that the best course for recovery from surgery is to get you up and moving about as quickly as possible. So on day two, I was up and moving, at least enough to shuffle to my door and back. However, as my strength increased, I was able to "race" my roommate down the hall. I'm sure that we looked like stereotypical geriatric patients in a full-care facility.

Over the course of my hospital stay, I enjoyed what seemed to be an endless stream of visitors, which was very pleasant, for the most part. By the second day, Debra had returned home to the job she had to maintain. But my dad was around, and he visited every day on his way home from work. And Debra had left me in the charge of my good friend, Dion, who also visited every day, just to make sure I was okay. In addition, I had a lot of friends in the city, having grown up and worked in Saskatoon, as well as having continued to spend summers there after leaving to study in Regina. However, since most of my friends and family had jobs, their visitation clustered around the late afternoon and evening. That made daytime one long, boring waiting period. You know you are bored when you anticipate mealtimes in a hospital, especially when that experience is reduced to merely wondering whether I would get any food at all and, if so, what flavour the Jell-o would be or what novel way there might be to prepare dry toast.

While there were precious few highlights to punctuate the monotony of my hospital recuperation, there were some memorable moments yet to come.

-10-

The Turtle

In the High and Far-Off Times the Elephant, O Best Beloved, had no trunk. He had only a blackish, bulgy nose, as big as a boot, that he could wriggle about from side to side; but he couldn't pick up things with it. But there was one Elephant—a new Elephant—an Elephant's Child—who was full of 'satiable curiosity, and that means he asked ever so many questions.

Rudyard Kipling, "The Elephant's Child" in *Just So Stories*

When I was a kid, I read a Dr. Seuss story called Yertle the Turtle. Of course, at the time, I did not know that it was about Adolph Hitler and his quest for world dominance; all I knew was that it was a cool story about a turtle and I loved his name. I have loved all things reptilian as long as I remember. A few years earlier, I had purchased an iguana as consolation for making a trip to see Sting in Edmonton, only to have the concert cancelled the day I arrived. I did not name my lizard Sting; I named him Bazyl, a tip of the hat to John Cleese and his Basil Fawlty character, as well as to the bass player from Blue Rodeo, Bazil Donovan, who had first gotten me thinking about alternative ways of spelling the name.

Of course, owning a lizard (six feet in length by that time) and a steady childhood diet of Dr. Seuss books caused me—most naturally, as they would anyone—to quite passionately want a turtle. Until that point, I had simply never gotten a proper opportunity to get one. Nonetheless, when Debra showed up in my hospital room on Friday evening, beaming brightly, with a small box in hand, there was no reason for me to connect the above pieces of information with the present moment. Instead, I logically thought, "That must be a model car or a piece of jewellery." Not once did I think, "My dear wife, out of her devotion to me, has brought an animal beloved to me into the hospital, here amongst the sick and dying, and, to wit, an animal known to carry all manner of diseases on its exterior, not the least of which is salmonella."

Such sober considerations led to my less than fully enthusiastic response to the small, beshelled creature with glinting eyes who looked up at me when I opened the box. I'm sure I was fully twice as startled by him as he was by me.

"Yikes! Get this thing out of here!"

I love my wife, and, until Yertle "ran" away, I loved my turtle. But sometimes even the best gift suffers from not being carefully thought through in its presentation.

-11-

Laughter, the Best Medicine

(except for when you have abdominal stitches and risk breaking
your gut open and spilling your insides all over the guy sitting in
the seat ahead of you)

*"Jack shall have Jill; Nought shall go ill;
The man shall have his mare again, and all shall be well."*

Puck to Lysander in William Shakespeare, *A Midsummer Night's Dream*

It was Sunday evening. Debra had returned to Regina, having spent a
lovely, turtly kind of weekend in the hospital with me, and I was on day
seven of my captivity. By this point, all my tubes had been removed,
except for the drain, that infamous tube running into the wound
site in my abdomen and capped on the exterior end with a bulb to
collect whatever waste the healing process was producing inside of me.
Although I had my appetite back and my strength was returning, the
nurse said I could not go home with this object still attached to me. A
compromise was struck: it was time for a night out on the town.

During my high school and early university years in Saskatoon, I
had discovered two entertainment sources which had provided much
laughter for my friends and me. First, there was the weekly improv
night at the Broadway Theatre, called the *Saskatoon Soaps*. With a story
line based on characters in a fictional high-rise apartment, the comedy
troupe kept us in stitches (no pun intended) in their hour-long romp
through an improvised script each Friday at midnight. Second, there
was *Shakespeare on the Saskatchewan*, a creative production put on by
another local troupe every summer in a big tent by the river's edge. The
dialogue stuck close to the Shakespearean original, but the settings
were novel. I specifically recall their production of Romeo and Juliet,
which toured Canada presenting the Montague family as English-
speaking and the Capulets as French—complete with fully bilingual
dialogue. (I thought of asking for half-price admission because I could

only understand 50% of what was said!) I also remember an excellent
rendition of *Othello*, which was set in pre-Confederation Canada,
where Othello was not a Moor, but rather a First Nations character,
played by Tom Jackson, a much-renowned Aboriginal actor. (Jackson
cuts an imposing figure and has long been the pride of Canada in music,
on stage, and in front of the camera. In my mind, he really came into his
own when he took a leading role in an episode of *Star Trek: The Next
Generation*.)

Back in the hospital where I awaited my night out, a few of my
friends had invited me to a performance of *A Midsummer Night's
Dream*. As the nurse issued my evening pass from lock-up, exacting my
promise to return that evening, she inquired as to where I might
be going.

"Going with some friends to a Shakespeare play."

"Which one?"

"*A Midsummer Night's Dream*."

"Comedy? I heard it was really funny. Don't forget your pillow!"

A few days earlier, one of my jailers (okay, care givers, but I did feel
as though I were in prison) had given me a pillow with the admonition,
"Your stitches are particularly fragile at this point. If you get the urge to
sneeze, be careful 'cause you could tear some of them out with violent
contractions. If you have to sneeze or cough, put this pillow across the
incision and hold tight. That will keep everything together."

I guess the nurse giving me my evening pass speculated that
laughing had the same potential to create harmful tension as did
sneezing or coughing.

Most of that play is now a blur at this distance, except for my vivid
memory of its intense comedic value. It was so funny that I was sure
that I was going to burst open my staples and explode right there in the
bleachers. Imagine the irony of a guy being "unseam'd … from the nave
to the chaps" in the middle of an audience at a Shakespearean comedy.
I think I missed half of the play because I was alternating between
uproarious laughter and clutching my pillow to my abdomen while
grinding my teeth in pain, trying to prevent my insides from becoming
my outsides.

Having survived the evening, and feeling fully refreshed from the
night out filled with friendship, laughter, and the occasional misgiving
that I'd have to be rushed back to the emergency, I tried to sneak quietly
back into my room. I had missed my curfew, which oddly enough had
the same feeling as coming home late when I was in high school: I'd get

into the house relieved that everyone was asleep, only to find my Dad sitting on the couch in his bathrobe, ready to confront me about where I'd been, whether I'd forgotten my watch at home, and where in the city I could have been that a phone had not been available. The night duty nurse was indeed at her post as I walked by the nursing station, and I heard, "Kind of late, isn't it?" My murmured "yes, mom" under my breath was followed by an audible "sorry" as I returned to my room.

-12-

Going Home

"No matter how dreary and gray our homes are, we people of flesh and blood would rather live there than in any other country, be it ever so beautiful. There is no place like home."

Dorothy in L. Frank Baum, *The Wonderful Wizard of Oz*

As with all good things, my incarceration at the hospital in Saskatoon eventually came to an end. On July 8th, just before I was discharged, I got a visit from Dr. Pfeifer, whose check-ins had become less and less frequent as my healing had progressed.

"Everything looks good, Dennis. I've consulted with CancerCare, and it looks as though there will be no requirement for any follow-up from their end, but I'll need to see you regularly, just to ensure that everything is healing and that this isn't coming back. So, I'm going to schedule you for a colonoscopy in six months, and then regularly from then on, at least for a few years."

"Okay."

Handing me his business card, Dr. Pfeifer said, "If you have any problems in the next few days, feel free to call me."

"Okay."

Debra had fully resumed her regular work life, having eked as much grace out of her employer as she could, so she was not even in town on the day I was released. However, Dion was there to pick me up, pack me up, and drive me the two and a half hours south to Regina. I've always been grateful for the generosity of good friends.

A friend of mine, Dave, once recounted the story of his first colonoscopy upon my telling him my story of 20 years ago. He spoke of the preparation and the procedure and then said, "My doctor said to me, 'If you experience an unusual amount of bleeding, call my office.'" At which Dave had mused to himself, "What is an unusual amount of bleeding? Wouldn't any bleeding be unusual?" He said nothing aloud, however, and failed to get any clarification from his doctor, simply proceeding home instead. Well, the surgeon had not fully cauterized a biopsy site created during the scope, and Dave did in fact begin to bleed. He explained to me, "I went to the bathroom and, whoosh, out comes a gush of blood. I began to feel a bit faint, so I went to my wife and, having told her what was happening, I asked, 'What should I do?' To which she responded, 'Get to the hospital, you idiot!'" (I am perhaps making her phrasing tamer than it was in real life). Dave subsequently spent a few days in the hospital recovering from what turned out to be too close a brush with death.

The day after I arrived home, I saw a few drops of blood in the toilet when I went to the bathroom. I was not really sure what to do. While I didn't want to panic, Dr. Pfeifer had not said anything to me about expecting bleeding, and I had no idea what was supposed to be normal. Not wanting to leave anything to chance, I gave his office a call.

"Could I please speak to Dr. Pfeifer? I'm experiencing a bit of bleeding."

"Just a minute, I will put you through to the operating room."

"Operating room?" I said—to myself, as I was already on hold. "No, no, wait! It can't be *that* important!"

"Hello. Dr. Pfeifer here."

"Dr. Pfeifer, this is Dennis Maione. Are you really in the middle of an operation? This can wait, I think."

"No problem; the nurse is holding the phone. How can I help you?"

"Well, I got a few drops of blood when I went to the bathroom this morning. Should I be worried about that?"

"No, not at all," he chuckled. "As the anastomosis heals, it will begin to squeeze the sides of your intestine a bit, and the wound will ooze. Do not worry unless you are seeing gushes of blood come out."

"Whew. Okay, sorry to have bothered you."

"Call me again any time; do not hesitate. Better to be safe than sorry."

"Thanks."

And so, my recovery began. It had been 14 weeks since I first entered a walk-in clinic to see about some bleeding that I was having, and now, seemingly, my cancer journey was over.

A month later, Debra and I went on a memorable summer vacation, including a day of mountain biking. I got stronger and stronger, finished school, and Debra got pregnant with our first child. Hope continued to spring eternal.

Colonoscopy

Inconvenience ... is only one aspect, and that the most unimaginative and accidental aspect of a really romantic situation. An adventure is only an inconvenience rightly considered. An inconvenience is only an adventure wrongly considered.

G.K. Chesterton, "On Running After One's Hat"
in *All Things Considered*

While I did not have to endure significant lifestyle changes due to my cancer and recovery, I was subjected to frequent follow-up and surveillance measures. This came in the form of regular visits to Dr. Pfeifer to "get scoped." The procedure, a colonoscopy, consisted of running a fibre-optic cable through my large intestine to check for colon health, specifically, to see if polyps—small growths forming on the intestinal wall—were forming. If a polyp is found, the scope also has the capability of removing, or *snaring,* it, after which the polyp is sent to the lab to work up to check for cancer. It can also biopsy suspicious-looking areas.

The good thing about the colonoscopy surveillance was the tremendous reassurance it provided to Debra and me. We learned that a tumour typically took about a decade to develop from the first cell abnormalities through the precancerous changes of a polyp to finally reach the stage of malignancy. My getting a regular scope made us both feel that I was far safer than the general population, who only received colonoscopies as a diagnostic step after they presented with problems to their physician. With a ten-year incubation time before real trouble could develop in my colon, I was well-protected against future malignancies. Any suspicious changes could be assessed far before then, and polyps, which posed the threat of becoming malignant, could easily be removed. There seemed to be no reason I should ever have to deal with colon cancer again. Precautionary procedures, yes, but malignancy appeared to be out of scope (pun noted). This confidence turned out to be misplaced, unfortunately, but I am getting ahead of myself.

I found the colonoscopy procedure itself rather cool because I got to watch on a monitor as the cable traversed my large intestine.

"That's the rectum; there's the anastomosis; into the sigmoid, now up the descending colon, across the transverse; hmmm, oh, that's just a bit of poop there; we can suction that out; down the ascending colon, and finally, the cecum, and we're all done."

It was the preparation for the procedure that was the killer.

CAUTION: What follows is a humorous but graphic account of colon prep; skip forward a few pages if you have a weak stomach—I'd hate to lose you this soon in the book!

Colonoscopies are the gold standard for the detection of tumours and polyps in the large intestine because they provide an opportunity for the surgeon to get a first-hand look at the intestinal wall, with the added convenience of providing a fast and efficient way to perform biopsies of tissue that looks suspicious. The problem, from the patient's perspective, is that the colon needs to be clean and free of all debris in order for the surgeon to do his job properly. This is so important that, if you have not done the cleaning properly, your surgeon may call off the procedure and reschedule it for a later time, as happened to me once.

Now, cleaning technologies and solutions have progressed a bit from when I had my first colonoscopy more than 20 years ago, although the general principle is still the same: create an environment in the large intestine wherein as much liquid as possible is directed internally, thus washing out all the contents and rendering the colon as clean as the proverbial whistle. This always involves ingesting, by mouth, some product robust enough to induce a gastrointestinal lavage. I think the word *lavage* is French for *firehose*, but I have never gotten confirmation of that.

I was sent the instructions for bowel preparation a few days before my first colonoscopy, and they read something like this:

(1) Purchase the gastrointestinal lavage, GoLYTELY, from a pharmacy.
(2) Prepare as directed.
(3) Drink 1 glass every hour until contents are consumed.
Note: For the 24-hour period from midnight to midnight on the day of preparation prior to the procedure, you may only drink clear fluids. After midnight the morning of the procedure, do not consume anything by mouth.

The day before the preparation was to begin, I visited the local pharmacist and asked for GoLYTELY. He nodded and returned with a four-litre jug which was empty except for a bit of powder at the bottom. With what must have been a perplexed look on my face, I paid for my purchase and took it home. The instructions were clear: fill the jug with water; shake; consume. Nothing could be hard about that.

Here is what I discovered. First, with no disrespect to BrainTree Laboratories, Inc., I think their product is misnamed. It should be called something like, "Go really heavily," or "Go until you think your internal organs are going to shoot out of you:" you get the idea. What I can say is that there was a lot of *go,* but no *lightly* at all. Second, drinking four litres of what amounted to expensive salt water is a lot more difficult than it seems. As the day progressed, just the thought of taking my next dose caused my mouth to water (the kind of watering that you experience just before throwing up). Thank you, B.F. Skinner, for identifying behavioural therapy; I am now completely cured of my desire to drink sea water.

By the end of the day, I was exhausted and hungry but internally cleansed. One unexpected benefit of this ordeal was that I discovered and learned to really love hot Jell-o. Having read that Jell-o qualified as one of the clear fluids I was allowed to ingest during the lavage (as do hard candies, Freezies, ginger ale, and chicken noodle soup without the chicken or the noodles—which Debra informs me is just called broth), I found myself wondering what the quickest form of delivery was. On the side of the Jell-o package, it says you can speed up the setting of the substance by adding ice to the hot water once the crystals have been completely dissolved. However, I was given pause by the idea that perhaps I could just drink it hot. What a revelation that proved to be! I will never eat solid Jell-o again.

The first follow-up scope I received was much as I remembered from my initial visit to Dr. Pfeifer in the hospital before my surgery. The only difference was a strange lump at the beginning of the journey: the anastomosis, I was told. Interestingly, Dr. Pfeifer took a couple of pictures of it and gave them to me, a memento of a trip to the nether world and back.

Once it was done, and Dr. Pfeifer had declared me free from cancer for the time being, I asked, "So, where did that cancer come from?"

"Well, beats me. If you were 60 and had been cooking over an open fire for 40 years, I might have some idea. But a 27-year-old getting this kind of cancer is extremely uncommon. If we could discover why, there might be a Nobel prize in it for the two of us."

Ironically, it had been only seven years earlier, in 1984, that Dr. Henry Lynch's work had uncovered a specific genetic condition that predisposed individuals to high rates of cancers, especially colorectal cancer, as well as uterine cancer in women. The condition was named hereditary nonpolyposis colon cancer (HNPCC), not because polyps are never involved, but to distinguish it from another genetic cancer syndrome, familial adenomatous polyposis (FAP), which typically involves hundreds of polyps. The name for HNPCC was later changed to Lynch syndrome when it was discovered that its defective gene was responsible for many other malignancies besides colorectal cancer. And indeed, it was Lynch syndrome that was the root cause of my early cancer—something I was not to discover until several more years down the road.

-14-

The Intervening Years
and Lynch Syndrome

*Until we understand the original dark, in which we have neither sight
nor expectation, we can give no hearty and childlike praise
to the splendid sensationalism of things.*

G.K. Chesterton, *Heretics*

Time and perspective mean everything when it comes to the way that
everyday occurrences are perceived. Later in this narrative, I will talk
about the tendency to see cancer everywhere, especially once my status
as carrier of a cancer-promoting mutation was discovered. However,
post-surgery, cancer was never prominent in my mind. Much of that
is because I'm not really a worrier, especially about things I can't
change. For Debra, it's a completely different matter. She worried
when I was diagnosed. She worried as surgery approached. She worried
during surgery. She continued to worry afterward. She loves me and
is concerned about my welfare. Usually, when it comes to me and my
health, I am unconcerned. And certainly I don't think about cancer
every time something unusual happens to my body. Cue intestinal
distress and explosive diarrhoea.

I don't know where it came from, but come it did, and it was
outrageous. One day, I was fine; the next, I was having explosive,
foaming diarrhoea. I thought, "Yuck, that is nasty; I should go see the
doctor." Debra thought, "Oh no, what if ..." and the word she could
not say.

Throughout the years, Debra has wept many tears over my cancer.
Some tears of sadness, others of joy, many of fear, and some bitter tears
over circumstance. And I can say that I still cannot fully appreciate
the depth of caring that produced those tears. I cannot appreciate the
terror in the night as she dreamt the death of her husband. I often
don't understand how her mind comes to conclusions, but I've come

to understand that her reasons are profoundly different from mine, and they bring a new and fresh perspective to my own experience. Sometimes this perspective is frustrating. Sometimes it makes me angry. But sometimes it humbles me to consider what the depth of her love drives her to.

She fears the spectre in the dark that I cannot fear because I do not see it, or I choose not to. And that fear she has in common with many many people.

So, in 1996, when I got giardia, a water-borne parasite, Debra saw cancer—especially when, after I'd submitted a faecal sample, the doctor's office phoned our home and left a message for me to call back. That scenario felt far too akin to the fateful summons we'd received in Regina four years earlier in order for Debra not to worry about impending doom. So, when I eventually arrived home and phoned the doctor back to find out it was giardia, Debra was ecstatic. Never before had anyone felt so overjoyed upon news of having a robust intestinal parasite. It was simple enough to diagnose and treat, and it was persistent enough that I had motivation to get it dealt with. My mind does not jump to cancer when I think about illness. Hers does. Maybe I'm psychologically better off for not obsessing about cancer, and maybe I'm alive because she does.

For the next decade or so, cancer faded from my mind, except for the regular scopes I had to endure: every six months for the first year, annually after that, and eventually every two years. In those years, Debra and I moved from Regina, to Toronto, to Edmonton, and finally to Winnipeg. On our last move, we took with us a substantially increased household: our children had all been born in Edmonton. After we had reached three children within the span of three and a half years, Debra stayed at home full-time and soon began homeschooling them. I worked, wrote books, and became a cyclically successful businessman (but that is a different book). Although I'd been making an annual trek from Edmonton to Saskatoon for scopes from Dr. Pfeifer, once we ended up in Winnipeg, we decided I should change surgeons because a 10-hour drive to Saskatoon for a regular medical test was impractical in the long term. So, it was a teary goodbye to Dr. Pfeifer, who had, literally and heroically, given me my life back. But with that goodbye came a new hello, to Dr. Cliff Yaffe, surgeon *extraordinaire*. That introduction was to come in September of 1999.

Dr. Yaffe picked up where Dr. Pfeifer had left off, scoping me every two years. In March of 2004, I had a scope, and, in his clinical notes, he remarked that my interval should be changed to five years: I had been free of cancer long enough to justify a relaxation in my surveillance. I'm not sure if he told me at that time; the anaesthetic I was given during my scopes always ensured that my short-term, post-scope memory was effectively obliterated.

But, in spring of 2004, everything changed for me. This came in the form of a phone call from my mother.

"Hello."

"Hello, Dennis!"

"Hi, Mom! How are things?"

"Fine. I want to let you know there's a letter coming in the mail to you from my genetic counsellor. I got a call from one of your cousins a few months ago. Like you, she had colon cancer, and of course you know that her mom, my sister, had uterine cancer, just as I did. She had colon cancer too, after that. Your cousin's doctor looked at the family history and thought she was a good candidate for a new genetic test for a condition called HNPCC. It turns out that she has it, and they think your aunt, who got multiple cancers and eventually died of one of them, must have had it too. As a result, they recommended the whole extended family be tested, and I came out positive. Given the bizarrely early onset of your cancer, it's more than likely you also have this gene, so you should get tested too."

"Really? Bad genes, eh? Well, at least that explains things. Given what you've just told me, I must have the same bad gene."

"Yeah."

A few days later, an official-looking package from my mother's genetic counsellor arrived in the mail. In it, a letter said she'd been diagnosed with a genetic syndrome called hereditary nonpolyposis colon cancer (HNPCC). It went on to say she had a variant of this syndrome called MSH2, an indication that her body fails to produce the MSH2 protein. The lack of this protein, one of several mismatch repair (MMR) proteins in the body, predisposes her to cancer. This is a dominant gene, so, if it had been passed on to me, I would manifest physical symptoms in keeping with it.

"Well, too late for this revelation," I thought. "A genetic test won't surprise me with its results."

I saw nothing urgent about jumping through the hoop of a genetic test, since I believed I knew what its pronouncement would be, so I just left it for a while. Opening the genetic can of worms, however, piqued my interest in the backstory, one much larger than I realized and full of drama that I never guessed at.

-15-

Prime Mover

There is something that comprehends them all, and that as something apart from each one of them, and this it is that is the cause of the fact that some things are and others are not and of the continuous process of change.

Aristotle, *Physics*

I am a religious man. At least, that is what my friends who are not church-going would call me. If you want to put a label on me, you might call me a quasi-conservative, evangelical Christian. Despite this, I can be a bit of a skeptic, and I don't jump quickly to seeing miracles and the hand of God. Jesus did not heal me from cancer—certainly not in the way that the stereotypical televangelist would like me to have been healed, with a smack on the head and a clean bill of health the next day (and perhaps some money in his pocket). Nonetheless, I am a firm believer in both mystery and science. And I am willing to believe that coincidence can sometimes be the mysterious manipulation of events by a deity who loves me and is actually interested in how my life turns out. Despite understanding the law of large numbers—that all statistical sets have outliers which defy the odds and thereby create seemingly mysterious and miraculous scenarios—I cannot help but see in my life and my journey a purposeful adjustment of my own circumstances and those of others around me.

As a result of my mom's revelation that a genetic mutation existed in my family, I became interested in how that information had first come to light. I learned that in December of 1999, my aunt had been diagnosed with colorectal cancer. In the spring of 2000, her daughter, my cousin Mona, had had a routine physical exam, in the course of which the subject of my aunt's colon cancer had come up. Mona describes the incident: "When I was talking to him that day and he asked about the cancer in the family, I told him about my mom. Then he looked at me silently for a long moment as if he was deciding what to do." Inexplicably, Mona's doctor had suggested she have a routine colonoscopy. This diagnostic procedure, performed on a physician's hunch, turned out to be pivotal in Mona's life, my personal journey, and those of the rest of my family. This procedure—an odd one to perform on a 38-year-old woman with no symptoms and with only her mother's cancer as any kind of red flag—ended up saving not only my cousin's life, but also those of many other members of my family over the years, including mine, and it will continue to do so in the years to come. Once again, Mona's words explain: "God whispered in his ear that day, and he listened, and sometimes that is all it takes."

Due to a cancellation, Mona was able to have a colonoscopy within two days. It revealed cancer: a tumour she was able to spot as she watched the colonoscopy image on the screen and suddenly noticed tissue that did not look normal. Through a series of further fortunate cancellations, she was recovering from surgery to remove her tumour only 14 days later.

Afterward, based on Mona's young age, her mom's cancers, as well as the bowel cancer I'd had at age 27 and my mom's cousin had had at age 23, Mona was referred to a genetic counsellor at the Tom Baker Clinic in Calgary. A detailed combing of the family tree to look for cancers turned up a significant number of similar malignancies in people of unusually young ages.

The genetic counsellor said, "I suspect there is a genetic component to the frequency and early onset of the cancers in your family, and we'd like to test someone. In order to ensure we test someone who is likely to have a genetic mutation, we'll do the test on you, Dennis, or your mom's cousin."

Mona volunteered to be the test subject, and her blood sample was sent to a lab in California for testing. It came back positive for one of the HNPCC (or Lynch syndrome) mutations, MSH2. Genetic counselling and testing were then offered to our whole family.

Western theology contains the concept of the prime mover, the mysterious and personal force who set everything in motion, the one who put the *bang* in the Big Bang Theory. However, prime movers can also be people in various circumstances in our lives, circumstances which are not generally religious or spiritual in nature. Mona's doctor was such a prime mover: because of his hunch, born for unknown reasons, a series of events were set in motion that culminated in revealing the cause of the cancers in my family. Often I wonder to myself who moved that prime mover.

-16-

Just When You Thought It Was Safe to Go Back in the Gene Pool

My scientific studies have afforded me great gratification; and I am convinced that it will not be long before the whole world acknowledges the results of my work.

Gregor Mendel, *The Proceedings of Brünn Society for Natural Science (1835)*

On January 11, 2006, I had a visit with Dr. Yaffe in his office. At this point, he had been doing a scope every two years, with an office visit in alternate years just to ensure that I was feeling well. He had finished a general physical examination of me, and, as we wrapped things up, the conversation turned this way: "Well, Dennis, you have been clear now for 13 years. I think it's time to change the surveillance interval from every two years to every five years. Congratulations."

"Excellent!" I exclaimed.

As I collected my things from the examining room, I said, in an offhanded way, "Hey, I'm not sure if this is important, but I got a call from my mom a few months ago. She said that she has something called HNPCC. Does that change things at all?"

Dr. Yaffe paused and then said, "Considerably, actually. I think we need to stick with a scope every two years. Protocol for HNPCC surveillance says every one to two years, but because you've been cancer-free for so long, I think it's safe to use the outside number, at least for now."

He paused again. "I think your experience bears out that you have an HNPCC gene; however, if you'd like, I can refer you to a geneticist to get a test done and confirm your status."

"Sure, let's do that."

So Dr. Yaffe sent a referral for genetic counselling and testing to Dr. Bernie Chodirker, a geneticist specializing in paediatric cases. On April

5th, 2006, I missed my appointment.

I saw Dr. Yaffe again on May 16th, when my newly reestablished biannual scope appointment came around. It was relatively clean: there was one small polyp that he removed, the second growth in the ascending colon that he had discovered over the past four years. Pathological testing in the lab showed that the tissue was benign, and I was given a clean bill of health once more.

A couple of months later, on July 12th, Debra and I were in the office of Dr. Bernie Chodirker on a matter regarding one of our children. In the course of the appointment, Dr. Chodirker said, "Dennis, I see you had been referred to me for genetic testing."

"Yes, my mom has an HNPCC mutation, and I'm supposed to get my blood tested to see if I have it too. I already know that I have it, though, since I had rectal cancer in my 20s. Dr. Yaffe gives me regular colonoscopies, but he figured I might want to know for sure one way or the other."

"So, your mother has HNPCC, does she? Which variant of the mutation does she have?"

"My mom has the mutation, yes, but I forget which variant she has."

"Are you Mennonite?"

"Well, yes, in fact; my mother is. Why do you ask?"

"There is a variant of this syndrome which is prevalent locally in the Manitoba Mennonite community. Because you don't know which variant you have, our general protocol is to test for that one first because it's a test we can do here in Winnipeg. If that comes back negative, we send the blood sample to Vancouver, where they can do more complete testing."

"Interesting."

"Is there some reason that you have been putting off this test?"

"Not really; I just never got around to it because, well, it did not seem an urgent thing to do. I'd like to do it now, though."

"Well, you can go directly to the lab, and we'll draw your blood and get it tested."

I was happy to get the deed done and went straight to the in-clinic lab.

As an aside, and in an ironic twist, the typical variant of Lynch syndrome in Manitoba Mennonites that Dr. Chodirker had suspected in me is MLH1, which is not the variant I actually have. I have MSH2. This identification of a cultural–religious group with a specific variant of the syndrome has caused more than a bit of trouble in my home province of Manitoba: for a while, one of the diagnostic questions for determining whether someone was eligible to get genetically tested under the province's health care program was, "Are you a Mennonite?" Things hit the proverbial fan on one occasion when a woman who met all the diagnostic criteria for Lynch syndrome, but who answered the final screening question with, "No, I am not a Mennonite," was denied testing solely because of that response. The medical community quickly realized that it was not only diagnostically but also politically incorrect to determine treatment eligibility based on religious or ethnic heritage.

To be fair to the medical establishment, they had set up the diagnostic criteria with both good intentions and fundamentally sound methodology; however, their approach simply lacked good optics and sufficient flexibility. It is indeed the case that genetic mutations tend to cluster within families and within cultural groups which have a predisposition to social isolation. In groups where the fear of religious or cultural contamination is significant, the gene pool becomes closed, so that when a genetic problem is introduced, it tends to be perpetuated. This happened in the 19th century to European royal families, the descendants of Queen Victoria, as they passed haemophilia around, and this phenomenon continues to happen around the world today.

So, having failed the Manitoba test for Lynch syndrome (my test having come back negative for the MLH1 mutation on September 21st), my blood was sent to Vancouver for more comprehensive testing. On May 24th, 2007, almost 10 months after my blood was drawn, the test came back positive for the MSH2 variant (oh well, I was not in a hurry anyway). I think it was around this time that I began to seriously consider the implications of a dominant genetic mutation for my children.

-17-

The Next One

Nothing is so painful to the human mind as a great and sudden change.
The sun might shine or the clouds might lower, but nothing could
appear to me as it had done the day before.

Mary Shelley, *Frankenstein*

The story is told of a man who, when flying, would always pack a bomb in his luggage. He had surmised that, while it was statistically unlikely there would be a bomb on any plane he flew on, the presence of two bombs on a plane would be so unlikely as to be effectively impossible.

Of course, the blunder our hapless traveller made was to assume the presence of his bomb had any effect on the chances that a terrorist would be present on his flight. He should have paid more attention in his statistics class.

Two cancers in the same person can either be related or unrelated. If they are unrelated, that person is essentially very unlucky, much like the guy who gets hit by lightning twice. Each separate but unrelated incidence is very unlikely; the occurrence of one, however, does not make the occurrence of another any more or less likely to happen. That is the definition of unrelated. And with cancer, every unrelated incidence is called a primary occurrence.

There are some people for whom two consecutive cancers are related. One set of people within this group get cancer, and, despite the best efforts of doctors to rid their bodies of malignancy, still have some remaining cancer cells, cells which go dormant and then stay inactive for a period of time (remission). Eventually, this cancer reasserts itself: it may seem to be a second cancer, but it is really just the first cancer coming back. The recurrence of cancer could be at the same site as the original tumour, or it could be in a new site, the cancer having metastasized and moved to another location in the body. This resurgence of a previously "cured" cancer accounts for the majority of related cancer incidences.

The people in a second and much smaller group, are those with unrelated cancers. For them, one cancer generally indicates an underlying cause which spells an increased likelihood of a second or even a third incidence. Outside of severe environmental factors, like asbestos or a source of radiation, such propensities are generally due to genetic factors. While genes don't actually cause cancer in most cases, defective genes typically inhibit one of the body's natural defence mechanisms that help prevent cancers from developing.

Genetically induced propensities towards cancer are called genetic syndromes, which are akin to playing the game of life with diabolically loaded dice: while the roll of a standard die has a one in six chance of coming up with any of the six numbers, a loaded die favours a particular number, which tends to get rolled more frequently. Despite displaying this higher rate of frequency, a genetic syndrome can be tricky to detect, requiring good communication, keen observation within family groups, and doctors who understand and are willing to test for these mutations. If people lack good information, they can't put the clues together, and the anomaly can go undetected. Even when all the signs are there, recent incidents have shown that some doctors still fail to grasp the significance of these mutations and, as a result, do not insist that their patients get tested.

When I first sought medical help to find out why I was bleeding, my doctor asked standard diagnostic questions, as did all the doctors who saw me during the process. And, of course, one of those questions was, "Is there a history of cancer in your family?" To which, in my naiveté, I always answered, "Not really; my mother had uterine cancer; that's all." However, the clues were staring me in the face; all I had to do was look.

My Mom's side of the family is Mennonite. *Mennonite* means different things to different people, but one thing it means to virtually everyone is a prominent focus on family and family history. In fact, I clearly remember childhood trips to Alberta to visit my aunt and uncle, when a standard activity after church was to go to the cemetery to visit the graves of relatives and family friends we had not been around to see buried. And although Mennonite culture was not strong in my household, I still learned to play what is jokingly called the "Mennonite game" with anyone I met who had a familiar Mennonite surname: Penner, Friesen, Peters, Reimer, Dyck, and so on. The game progresses predictably.

"Mr. Dyck, do you have any relatives from the Rosemary, Alberta area of the country?" I might ask.

"Why yes, my mother's second cousin once removed was from there. Why do you ask?"

"Despite my having an Italian last name, my mother is from a Mennonite family, some of whom are still in the Rosemary–Brooks area."

At that point, we would begin tracing our family trees to see where they might intersect.

One might think, given my inherited cancer syndrome, that there would have been evidence in the family tree for me to have anticipated it. And indeed there was—plenty of it—except that I'd been oblivious to it. All I had ever been aware of was my mom's uterine cancer, and that had seemed as far from a personally menacing event as possible. Upon eventually consulting with one of the family historians, however, I found disturbing information in the family tree.

I didn't have to look past my grandmother to see the assertion of an autosomal dominant gene (one that manifests itself in any carrier and does not discriminate between men and women). Statistically speaking, the dominance of a cancer gene means that 50% of the children in a family with one parent as a carrier will inherit that gene, creating the increased likelihood of cancer, which would appear not only more frequently but also at an earlier age than in the regular population.

That is exactly what I found. The dice were loaded. My grandmother had cancer. She had five children, and three of those five had cancer, one of them being my mother. In turn, half of the kids of my grandmother's afflicted children got cancer, including me. And now, in my own family of three children, one son has the defective gene.

So the law of large numbers can be seen writ small in my familial group. And this is only amongst my first- and second-degree relatives. The same prevalence can be seen within the families of my grandmother's 10 siblings. And, while I had the distinction of being the youngest amongst my first- and second-degree relatives to get cancer, my mother's cousin got colon cancer at the age of 23, several years earlier than I did, so he gets the prize for youngest in the clan.

In addition to my discovering this gritty reality of the family tree (our "genetic *cess*pool," as one of my aunts, herself afflicted, likes to quip), my geneticist, Dr. Chodirker, did a thorough job of educating me on the specific statistics associated with Lynch syndrome. There are elevated rates of colorectal, uterine, stomach, breast, ovarian, small bowel (intestinal), pancreatic, prostate, urinary tract, liver, kidney, bile (gallbladder) duct, brain, central nervous system, and skin cancer occurrence in those affected by the Lynch mutation. The brutal truth continues: some of those elevated rates are in the double digits. Colorectal and uterine cancer rates are as high as 80% and 60% respectively. At least the majority of that long list of cancers occur at rates under 10%. When cancer does occur, it is often at a younger age than is normal: an average of age 45 for colorectal cancer, for example, as opposed to age 72 in the general population. The invaluable advantage of knowing such hard truths is that surveillance regimens can be put into place to catch cancers early, and even to detect precancerous cell changes.

Given that the list of Lynch cancer susceptibilities Dr. Chodirker had recently spelled out seemed to cover more body parts than it left out, Debra can be forgiven for reacting with concern one day at my casual mention of an abdominal pain. In June of 2007, I had begun feeling a mildly odd sensation on the right side of my abdomen. Despite living in a land of socialized medicine (or perhaps because of that), I am not one to cause stress to the medical system over things that are trivial, so I shrugged off my symptoms and carried on. After I eventually mentioned it to Debra, however, she suggested I see the doctor, and, thankfully, I complied.

I made an appointment to see our family physician, Dr. Doris Kyeremateng (many call her Dr. Doris).

"How can I help you, Dennis?"

"It's nothing, really. Just feeling a bit of abdominal pain."

Upon further questioning and examination, Dr. Kyeremateng announced, "It doesn't seem as though it's anything problematic, but given your history, I think we should get this checked out." She knew of my previous cancer as well as my newly diagnosed genetic status.

"Sure."

A couple of months later, after I'd forgotten all about it, I got notification in the mail that I was supposed to report for a CT scan on October 5th. I was confused, but after mulling things over, it dawned on me that this was the scan Dr. Kyeremateng had talked about scheduling when I'd last been in her office. I now thought this was all a bit of an overreaction, especially since the intestinal pain had effectively gone away. As I recall, I almost phoned to cancel, but things in my life were so busy that I never got around to it. When the day for the test arrived, I found myself wandering the halls of the hospital in yet another gown that closed in the back, following the mostly faded yellow line in search of the CT room.

I didn't think very much about the scan in the week that followed; in fact, it had pretty much gone out of my mind. So on Friday, October 12th, when Debra arrived at our office to pick me up from work, I was anticipating a quiet Thanksgiving weekend—the last before we were to leave for San Diego in a matter of days on a week's vacation. However, nothing would be further from the truth. As I prepared to leave, Debra plugged in her cell phone, which had been nonfunctional all afternoon due to a dead battery. I was in another room when I heard her call out in consternation, "Hey, my phone shows Dr. Kyeremateng called 15 times!" It seemed Debra's cell phone was the contact number we had given for all communication with our family. We soon found out that Dr. Kyeremateng had also called Debra's sister to see if there was some way she could get hold of us: Debra had a couple of messages from Colleen as well.

At 3:30 in the afternoon on that Friday, when I called in to my physician's office, I already knew I had cancer. Of course, it was the receptionist I spoke to, and I was told nothing on the phone—simply asked to come down right away. This, despite the imminent closing hour of the doctor's office. I remember watching Debra get into the passenger's seat of our van as I walked around to the driver's side.

"It's cancer," I said to her.

She nodded, lips compressed. The rest of the 15-minute trip was spent in silence, each of us alone with our thoughts and unspoken dread. Suddenly, our entire world hung suspended. Just like that, we had re-entered "the zone" which we'd so dearly hoped never to cross into again; the zone which, mere moments earlier, had been but a remote and barely recalled memory. Being propelled into this ugly territory now felt rudely and aggressively familiar, like a long-forgotten nightmare suddenly revived and staring at us eyeball to eyeball. The element of the surreal swirled around us, all the while feeling hideously real and immediate.

In the doctor's office, we were ushered immediately into an examining room. Dr. Kyeremateng arrived.

"I'm sorry to tell you: the CT scan showed a mass on your large intestine, in the cecum. That's at the beginning of the large intestine, just next to the appendix and across from the opening to your small intestine. I'm going to forward this result to Dr. Yaffe's office, and he will pick it up from there."

"Is it cancer?"

"You can't tell definitively from the scan, but it does appear to be. The diagnostic report says that it is 'consistent with a carcinoma.' Dr. Yaffe will have to determine what he wants to do in terms of definitive diagnostics, but the standard procedure would be to do a colonoscopy with a biopsy, so that a pathologist can look at actual tissue to make a final determination."

"Okay."

No tears this time as Debra and I left the doctor's office. We knew the drill; we were steeling ourselves for the weeks and months ahead. We knew what we were in for: at least, we thought we did.

But things were not the same as they had been the first time. Genetics, children, family business, second primary occurrence. These were some of the complicating factors we started to run into very quickly. The journey ahead was much longer and more arduous than we were prepared for.

It had been 15 years, 3 months, and 14 days since cancer had been removed from my body. 5,584 days since my abdomen had been violated by the cut of a scalpel searching for the villain amidst the blood. And on that day, the sign reading, "5,584 days cancer-free," came down and was replaced with one reading, "This body is out of order, again."

-18-

Providence, Coincidence, and the Law of Large Numbers

We see a universe marvelously arranged, obeying certain laws, but we understand the laws only dimly. Our limited minds cannot grasp the mysterious force that sways the constellations.

Albert Einstein (1929)

What elapsed over the next 24 hours were events about which Sheldon from *The Big Bang Theory* might say, "This would be one of those circumstances that people unfamiliar with the law of large numbers would call a coincidence."

The first event started out as a distraction, but it ended up being an occasion that would change, maybe even save, my life. On our way home from seeing Dr. Kyeremateng, Debra and I talked calmly, but we felt shell-shocked. I was driving. Debra used her cell phone to call our good friends, John and Wendy Botkin, who have always sustained us with their wisdom and stalwart friendship. She spoke with Wendy, who, along with John, received our bad news with deep dismay. Then, in typical Botkin fashion, they reached out to support us, inviting us to their home for the evening to join them for wine, cheese, and conversation with a mutual friend who was their houseguest, in town for a medical conference.

Pausing in her conversation with Wendy, Debra said to me, "John and Wendy want us to come over. For wine and cheese."

"Because I have cancer?" I exclaimed, teasing.

Overhearing me, Wendy sputtered on the other end of the phone and then answered, "Well, yes!" and it was settled: cancer party!

In the fall of 2007, I had three different phone numbers for Dr. Yaffe. The consulting company I operated was in the middle of a project for the Department of Surgery at the University of Manitoba, and Dr. Yaffe was in charge of the residency program for General Surgery at that time, so I had been working closely with him in a professional capacity. Rather than simply wait for him to receive information from the family doctor the following week, I decided to take matters into my own hands. After a few phone calls, though, I discovered he was out of town until the following week, so it seemed I would have to wait after all. I was content to send him an email, one with a subject line that read, "Need to talk with you asap ... looks like I'll need your services in short order."

Arriving at the Botkins' home a couple of hours later, we were grateful for their warm hospitality. There was graced conversation with John and Wendy and our mutual friend, Dr. Marilyn White: unlike the walrus and the carpenter, however, we never arrived at the more standard wine-and-cheese topics of shoes, ships, and sealing-wax. Instead, we talked of cancer, the advances in treatment options since the last time I'd had it, and the doctors in my life, now and to come. Marilyn spoke highly of Dr. Kyeremateng, whom she'd taught family medicine to. She also recommended an oncologist of high repute, Dr. Smith. We talked about reasons to be hopeful.

Marilyn would come to figure importantly in how my future played out, but the most significant role would be played by her husband, Dr. Rob James, PhD, whose expertise she also offered that evening. None of us, however, could have anticipated the drama that would eventually unfold and catch us all up.

While Rob will be mortified to find himself so prominently featured in my narrative, I can say with confidence that my life and treatment would have been drastically altered, for the worse, were it not for his wisdom and prodigious, relentless effort on my behalf as we wended our way through a labyrinth of treatment plans and options. He has characterized his role simply as "one of the many voices," but I can say that, outside of Dr. Yaffe, whose significant role will become apparent, Rob was the most important of our counsellors in the six months that followed that auspicious meeting, a role he continues to fulfill to this day. And, while I do have a vast array of people in my support community, as Rob likes to note, it is the case that some of these individuals have an identifiable influence which is both profound and disproportionate.

So, through the convergence of wine and friends and renewal of acquaintance, this phase of the journey was off to a good start.

The second event, which happened the following day, was not to be as life-changing, but, on its surface, was far more coincidental than the first.

In the years between my first and second diagnoses, my best friend, Dion—the same one who had cared for me in Saskatoon during my first hospital stay—had gone to medical school and become a vascular surgeon. By 2007, he had moved from Winnipeg, where he'd studied under Dr. Yaffe, and set up a practice in Nova Scotia. I remember going down to our laundry room (mundane chores still needing to be done in the midst of crisis) and giving him a phone call.

"Hello."

"Hey buddy, how are things?"

"Den! Good, how are you?"

"Well, it looks as though I have cancer again."

(A brief pause.) "Tell me about it."

I explained the lead-up, the CT scan, and the conversation I'd had with my family doctor.

"Wow, that's hard. But you cannot always believe the CT. What looks like a mass could just be faecal material in your intestine. Colonoscopy is still the gold standard for diagnosis."

"Yeah, well, I tried to call Dr. Yaffe, but he's out of town, so I'm waiting for him to get back to me to talk about the next steps."

Dion laughed, "He's actually right here in my living room. Would you like to talk with him?"

"What! Why is he there? Sure, put him on."

"He's here for a conference. Just dropped by my place to say hi. I'll put him on."

"Dennis! What can I do for you?"

"It seems I need your services, doc. A CT scan showed a mass on my large intestine: probably cancer."

"Well, let's do a colonoscopy and then take it from there. Call my office on Monday, and they can schedule something right away. Didn't we just do a scope?"

"Yeah, last year."

"Wow, it was clean then. This tumour appeared quickly."

After hanging up the phone, I marvelled at the unlikely events I had just experienced. While I *am* familiar with the law of large numbers, I still choose to see these happenings as acts of providence, the hand of a loving God in my life.

-19-

Decisions

I shall be telling this with a sigh
Somewhere ages and ages hence:
Two roads diverged in a wood, and I—
I took the one less traveled by,
And that has made all the difference.

Robert Frost, *The Road Not Taken*

Debra and I never did travel to San Diego. Instead, on October 24th, 2007, I had my last colonoscopy. Sure enough, I had cancer.

Getting cancer in the same place and for the same reason makes some things easier to do the second time. Calling my parents and the rest of my family was not as difficult. They had been through this with me the first time, and my having lived cancer-free for 15 years provided a lot of hope for my prognosis the second time around. I thought that I knew what to expect as well, and, fundamentally, I did, at least for the mechanics of the preparation and the surgery.

However, there were a lot of hard things associated with my second diagnosis and subsequent treatment. The first was my children. At the time of my first cancer, I'd had no kids. However, in the intervening years, we'd had a girl and two boys. In the fall of 2007, our children were 14, 12, and 10. Believing my confidence would provide a measure of reassurance to them, Debra and I sat down to tell them what was happening.

"We've told you about the cancer that I had before you were born and about the genetic condition I have that caused it. Well, I have cancer again. And I'll have to have surgery to get rid of it. I've been through this before, though, and there's nothing to worry about. But you need to know what's going to happen."

(Nods all around.)

"But Dad, people die from cancer," declared Alex, my middle child.

That was the moment I realized everything had in fact changed.

This was the first time I'd had a face-to-face encounter with someone who had no concept of probability or prognosis regarding my cancer, someone who did not share my confidence. My son was facing the possibility (in his mind, perhaps probability) that his dad could die from cancer.

Throughout the diagnosis, treatment, and follow-up of my initial cancer, there had never been a mention of death. Although Debra had feared its distant spectre, I had never glimpsed even the faintest shadow. Everything was relatively easy and matter-of-fact. Once I'd settled on Dr. Pfeifer as my surgeon, I had anticipated only surgery, recovery, and, in the worst case scenario, lifestyle changes as a consequence of treatment. But there would be no death. And, my expectations had been borne out in exactly this way. There had been nothing to worry about, and the only lasting effect had been a scar on my abdomen and a "six-pack" that would never be quite the same.

While my expectations were still the same, my son had not shared my earlier experience. Moreover, he was young and impressionable. So, we cried a bit together, my kids, my wife, and I, but, in the end, we all knew that everything would be okay. However, that initial encounter proved to be the harbinger of more struggle and complexity to come.

Something was different this time. In the follow-up appointment with Dr. Yaffe, he let me know that I had a choice to make regarding my treatment.

"We know that your tumour has been caused by your Lynch syndrome, so you have to decide what you want me to do. One course of action would be to do a hemicolectomy, a standard resection as Dr. Pfeifer did. Alternatively, and what I recommend, is that we do a total colectomy. This would essentially remove your entire large intestine, and I would attach what remains of your rectum to your small intestine. Technically, you would be left with an ileorectal anastomosis. By removing your large intestine, I would be removing the primary seat of cancer resulting from your genetics. While the large intestine is not the only place that Lynch cancers occur, it is, by far, the most common site. This is the closest thing to a cure for what you have."

"What are the implications for my lifestyle?"

"Your large intestine does nothing but remove liquid from your waste. There is very little nutrient absorption that goes on there. So, your stool will be looser than it was, and you will have to go to the toilet more often. In addition, I would have to remove the ileocecal valve, the natural regulator of flow between your small and large intestines. This would mean that the desire to go to the bathroom will come upon you more quickly than it used to. However, your body will adapt, and many of these things will normalize over time."

"How soon do I have to decide?"

"Any time before the surgery."

"I don't know ... I'm not sure. I'll have to think about this."

I went home and shared this startling information with Debra. Initially, I was strongly inclined to go with a hemicolectomy, something that I initially told Dr. Yaffe I wanted to do—essentially repeating the same procedure as the first time round, excising only the cancerous piece of my colon. For one thing, I was now operating a small business and dealing with more than a little concern about the length of time a colectomy would keep me away from earning a living. For another, I was feeling protective towards the body I had known and inhabited my entire life. I wanted to keep all of my body parts, not give up a major organ. After all, I was willing to undergo any surgery that would be required should another tumour surface in the next 15 years—which I was suddenly confronting as all too real a possibility. And if that was a price worth paying to avoid metastasized cancer, it was a price equally worth paying to retain my large intestine, I thought. (It's amazing how quickly you can become very emotionally attached to something you've essentially ignored your entire life, the moment you are threatened with its imminent removal. In the space of hours or less, I'd suddenly grown decidedly fond of my "four miles of tubing," as Peter Cook so aptly put it.)

While I was willing to entertain the prospect of serial surgeries, Dr. Yaffe had counselled a colectomy. And I couldn't ignore the fact that my body kept turning against me. Once again, I turned to my friend and advisor Dion, phoning him 3000 kilometres away to wrestle over the questions with me. Like Dr. Yaffe, Dion was of the opinion that I should opt for the colectomy. I objected.

I can remember saying, "All I really want to know is whether I can go canoeing with my boys and not have to stop every 500 metres to go to the bathroom."

Dion was sympathetic but realistic. "I cannot give you any guarantees. Everyone is different. But, what are you going to do, man— have a new surgery every time you get another tumour?"

"Yes," I announced, explaining my reasons. It turned out the situation was more complex than I'd suspected, however. What I hadn't fully thought through, and what Dion explained, was that surgery and recovery would become increasingly difficult as I aged. While I had weathered it well in my 20s, and hoped and expected to do so again now, repeated major abdominal surgery was not a thing to be considered lightly. With every decade I aged, and with every subsequent surgery—perhaps at shorter intervals than the one I'd experienced this time—there was the issue of increasing scar tissue making surgery more difficult. Not to mention the Russian roulette factor: clearly there were no guarantees, no matter what surveillance regimens might be in place, that future cancers would be found in a timely fashion and effectively contained.

I became increasingly perplexed, finding myself enmeshed in a dilemma far deeper than I'd anticipated. I think it was at this point Debra and I entered "research mode," and I believe we have never since relinquished any of that desire—perhaps compulsion—to find things out for ourselves. I started to make phone calls to try to figure out how I should proceed. What I quickly discovered is that there were virtually no people in my situation. The conversation I had with a nurse at an intestinal health clinic in Winnipeg was indicative of that.

"Hi. I'm hoping that you can give me some guidance," I said to the person who took the phone call. "I have colon cancer, and my surgeon is suggesting he remove my whole colon and attach my small intestine to my rectum. Can you tell me anything about the quality of life I might have afterward and about the length of time to recover?"

"We have a number of patients whom we've counselled and helped through this kind of procedure. Let's see. I had a patient who was able to return to work after about nine months. I also had a patient, a student, who was able to return to part-time studies after about five months of recovery."

"Five months?" I asked incredulously. "Nine months? That long? Wow!"

"Of course, everyone is different. How sick are you now?"

"I'm not sick at all. I feel fine. Why do you ask?"

"Oh, well, most of the patients I deal with have long-term chronic issues with their intestines, either Crohn's disease or ulcerative colitis. They are very sick, and the removal of their colons is a treatment of last resort. That is not you?"

"Not at all. Except for the tumour, there's nothing wrong with me at all. I've never felt better."

(A pause on the end of the line.) "I'm not sure I can help you much then."

I talked to a couple of general surgeons whom I knew, and there was not much help there either. It seemed to be very uncommon to remove a colon from a young person experiencing good health. As a result, not one person could give me a good indication of what my quality of life was going to be should I go ahead with it. So, to start my *pros* and *cons* list in making my decision, all I had on the *cons* side was *unknown*. However, the *pros* side was little better: all that was really clear to me was that removing my entire large intestine would probably reduce the chance I would get cancer again.

In the end, I decided to have my whole large intestine removed. The deciding factor was the idea of having this radical surgery while I was reasonably fit and healthy, as opposed to anticipating the same thing 15 years down the road when I would be less able to recover from and adapt to such a major shock.

So, having made the major decision, it was time to wait, again, for the date of surgery.

The Second Surgery

*"I could tell you my adventures—beginning from this morning," said Alice
a little timidly: "but it's no use going back to yesterday, because I was a
different person then."*

Lewis Carroll, *Alice's Adventures in Wonderland*

On November 9th, 2007, I checked into the hospital for surgery to
remove my large colon, including its 4.5 cm mass, and to connect my
small intestine (ileum) to what remained of my rectum. Unlike the first
time, I did not check in the day before, and I had to do the preparation
of intestinal cleansing myself. Moreover, I was not the same person I
had been 15 years earlier when I'd checked in for the same procedure.
In fact, given that, at 265 pounds, I was nearly 75 pounds heavier, I
was almost two new people. (That, and my subsequent recovery from
obesity, is a different story for another time.) On the other hand, I
had more life experience and carried more responsibility than before. I
also had more confidence: confidence that I would once again survive
this ordeal and come out whole on the other side (minus my colon, of
course).

I arrived with Debra at St. Boniface Hospital at 6:15 that morning,
and I was ushered into a room where I changed into my hospital garb.
Then I moved into a waiting room. My pastor, Al, and my friend, John,
were there, and we talked and prayed together as I waited. My surgery
was scheduled for 10:00 a.m., so I had a bit of time to kill, although it
ended up being considerably more than I was expecting. At about 8:30
a.m., an orderly came into the waiting room and explained there would
be a delay.

"It appears things are going to be held up for a couple of hours. An
elderly gentleman was just checked in through emergency, and Dr. Yaffe
has to do the surgery."

"Drat! Curses to you, anonymous old man who delayed my surgery
and may be responsible for my cancer progressing to an inoperable state

while I wait!"

I think that would have been what I thought, or even said, had I not been so tired. However, what I actually said was, "Okay."

After I'd sat a couple of more hours in the waiting room, an orderly finally arrived. He had me sit down in a wheelchair, and, after I got a hug and kiss from my wife, I was off.

I'm sure this orderly got training in perambulating hospital conveyances from the same fellow who had pushed me around at my first surgery. In fact, I believe there's an orderly school (*for* orderlies, not describing the way it's run)—probably in the Philippines, given the disproportionate number of Filipino orderlies I've had the pleasure to meet—where they teach them how to smile continuously, talk non-stop, and navigate hospital corridors as though they're drunken university students. We raced to an awaiting gurney and then to the pre-op room. At that point, I got the requisite intravenous line put in and was moved into the operating theatre.

I'm not sure why, but the room felt much more ominous to me than it had for my first surgery. I think it was largely because Dr. Yaffe was not in the room, and he was essential to the activity yet to begin. As a result, I got in a lot more thinking about where I was and what was about to happen. The walls were glaring white, the environment so sterile. One guy, whose role I did not know, talked incessantly about his cabin and plans to install new cabinets. I think he was there just to keep my mind off the wait, but it didn't work. I was feeling very cold and exposed on the operating table. My arms were stretched out, as though I were an insect being prepared for pinning to a specimen board. I found myself dreading the procedure to come and feeling afraid.

When Dr. Yaffe arrived, however, the atmosphere changed completely. It was comforting to hear a friendly and familiar voice telling me the names of all the people there and what their roles were; to listen to him tell everyone, as he did every time he performed a procedure on me, who my previous surgeon was, why I was there for surgery, and that I had HNPCC. To this day, every time I am with Dr. Yaffe for a procedure, he still begins with, "This is Dennis. He has HNPCC. His first surgeon was Joe Pfeifer in Saskatoon," a tribute to my past medical practitioner but also to Dr. Yaffe's own intrinsic desire to be a teacher in all circumstances. That is all I remember, as shortly afterward I was given anaesthetic and slipped into unconsciousness.

-21-

Hospital Recovery

*It is not ... that these are not quite well in body, but that they are not
quite used to being well; just as even a tranquil sea will show some ripple,
particularly when it has just subsided after a storm. What you need,
therefore, is .. confidence in yourself and the belief that you are
on the right path ... .*

Seneca, *The Stoic Philosophy of Seneca: Essays and Letters*

Recovery from surgery version 2.0 progressed physically much the same
as version 1.0 had. After the first day, they had me up to walk around
my room, and soon they were encouraging me to move about the ward.
Some things were different, however, both because treatment varied a
bit and because Debra and I had planned more this time around, having
had a better sense of what was to come.

I came out of surgery with fewer tubes than the first time. No
drain, no catheter, no central line. Instead, just the NG tube and an IV
in my arm. The incision site was larger than before, because a lot more
tissue had had to be removed. Dr. Yaffe had begun at the bottom of
the original incision, followed it up, and then extended it towards the
breastbone, effectively doubling the length of incision from the
first time.

More forethought had been put into my recovery period in
hospital. First, I had a television in my room. This was especially useful
as it was CFL (Canadian Football League) playoff time, and my team,
the Saskatchewan Roughriders, was progressing handily towards the
Grey Cup championship. The first weekend boasted the semi-finals, and
the Riders won their contest—although my drug-induced haze meant
the games I watched were a bit of blur to me. I had not been so high at
a football game since the year my dad and I had season tickets to the
Riders, sitting behind a group of guys who sat in a perpetual cloud of
pot smoke.

Second, we set up a plan for remembering my visitors. I cannot overstate the value of visitors during recuperation, at least in controlled bursts. Because days are so long when you sit in discomfort for hours on end, sometimes in a fog of painkillers that limits your ability to read or focus, having visitors to break up the boredom and to help engage your brain is of inestimable value. So, Debra created a visitor's book for me. We had a vast number of coloured pens so people could choose their favourite to write, doodle, or draw their greetings. All who visited were asked to write in the book and allow their pictures to be taken, so that I could remember the kindness of friends and family. Any cards they brought were also taped into the book.

There were too many meaningful moments during my time in the hospital to fully do justice to them. My kids showed up, and I explained what all the things in the room were and what everything did. Debra's parents, Henry and Eleonore, visited a number of times, stopping in to say hi and see how my recovery was progressing. My step-mother, Lori, came down from Saskatoon, and, besides spending time with Debra and me, spent some very special times with our kids, their memories including pizza, card games, and an overnight stay in the hotel. The kids bonded with their grandmother over copious amounts of food and their first football experience, watching the Roughriders win their semi-final game, a highlight that cemented their status as lifelong Riders fans (as Canadian readers will know, once a Riders fan, always a Riders fan).

My friends stopped by, cheering me with smiles, words of encouragement, and gifts (highlighted by the Saskatchewan Roughriders hat from John, which took me right through the semi-finals and their Grey Cup victory). My friend, Mike, summed up the position of the general group when he visited one day. We'd gone for a bit of a "jog" down the hallway, and upon my sitting down for a rest at the turn-around point, he said, "You're going to be okay, right? Because I consider you one of my good friends, and it would be inconvenient if you died." I laughed at the uncharacteristically effusive expression of love and caring.

On the home front, other significant things were happening. Debra's aunt drove from the opposite end of the city to pick up our dirty laundry, later returning it freshly cleaned and folded—with the gift of a casserole, to boot. In fact, food poured in from everywhere: Debra's mom and sister frequently delivered meals and treats, and fellow church members from the care group in our area took turns cooking for us. These actions all nourished our souls even more than our bodies (well, my body couldn't yet benefit from the food, unfortunately). Beyond simply heart-warming, the expressions of love we experienced were soul-supporting. There were cards and emails from one end of the country to the other, and prayer, once again, was going up all around the world. One woman in our church pledged to pray for me daily over an entire year and regularly sent me cards, notes, and wee gifts during that time.

There were moments of black humour as well. The morning Dr. Yaffe came into the room, for example, and, motioning to an article on the front page of the *Winnipeg Free Press*, told me I should get well soon or they'd be sending me out into the street, a reference to the decreasing length of time that hospitals in Canada were tolerating for patient recovery. Or the morning after a night of nausea, when, remembering someone's comment about acid reflux, I'd asked the duty nurse, "What does acid reflux feel like?" just before throwing up a stomachful of black bile into my lap. I always was one to try to save others inconvenience: this way, the nurse was right there; she wouldn't have to make a second trip to change my ... everything.

Third, taking full advantage of technology and the new trend towards social networking, Debra managed an Internet page she'd set up on a site called Carepages. These were the days before Facebook had attained the popularity it enjoys today, as well as the days before smartphones and ubiquitous wifi. She used a public computer in the cafeteria area to post updates to my Carepage directly from the hospital and so was able to bring my experience (and hers) into the lives of friends, families, and acquaintances, especially those who were not able to make the trek to Winnipeg to visit me.

In a truly ironic twist in my recovery, I was placed in a two-person room. My roommate, an older gentleman with whom I never did have a conversation, turned out to be the same person who'd been responsible for having bumped my surgery to a later time. Unfortunately, he brought with him a measure of incontinence that I had not experienced since my children had been babies. This full-scale, frequent, and unannounced bowel evacuation made life in that room almost intolerable. This worsened as the days progressed, both as the fog of my pain killers cleared and as I became increasingly irritated at my inability to recover sufficiently to go home. Debra recalls dreading her many exits from the elevator, her nose already detecting the odour that grew stronger as she turned the corner into my hallway. Whenever my roommate was absent, I would implore the nurses to find some solution to my problem. There was nothing much they could do except to move him into the hallway whenever they could. Debra bought a small bottle of air freshener at the hospital store in an attempt to alleviate my misery; however, all it accomplished was to create a pungent smell of heavily polluted strawberry. To this day, I experience waves of nausea every time I smell artificial strawberry. Fortunately, my roommate was released a few days before I was, so I got to spend the last three or four days alone and scent-free in the room.

Living at the mercy of others is a hard place to be in. I think one of the reasons for our fear of illness is the dread of giving up our self-determination and having to release ourselves into the care of others. For some, this is such a terrifying prospect that they would rather take their own lives than endure the ignominy of being cared for by others. For me, it was a hard balance between trying to be self-sufficient as I healed and recognizing my own limitations. There were many occasions over the last few days in hospital when I lay in my own vomit or waste and sighed as I called for a nurse to come and clean me up. On those occasions, I realized there is a thin line between humility and humiliation. And, for the length of time I stayed the proud, strong patient, my humiliation remained at the forefront of my experience. The essence of humility is being able to let go of pride and to embrace instead the comfort that can come only from others.

On the day before my release, two things happened that turned my mind from depression to hope. The first was a chance encounter with Dr. Yaffe in the hallway. At that point, he no longer visited me every day, for I was beyond the realm of what he could do for me, and my recovery care was really in the hands of the nurses. So, it had been a couple of days since I'd last seen him. I was doing my morning shuffle down the hallway, head down, tired of the sounds and nauseated by the smells of the hospital, and contemplating the possibility that I would never, ever, get out of that place. I looked up, and there he was. Now, Dr. Yaffe is an imposing man at any time: tall, stockily built, with a deep booming voice. At that time, he looked as though he were a giant. I caught his eye, and he said to me.

"Dennis, how are you feeling?"

"Awful, doc. I just want to go home."

I am sure there was more emotion in my voice than I wanted to communicate. In response, he put his hand on my shoulder and said, "It's going to be okay."

Something happened with those words. I'm not sure why, but

something happened. Here was my doctor, a man with years of training and many more years of experience. A man who was at the top of his field in Manitoba and across Canada. He did not offer me medical wisdom or a treatment plan. He offered me nothing more than a touch and words of hope, "It's going to be okay."

I think that was the turning point in my hospital recovery, more psychological than physical. That, coupled with the nurse who told me to "get off my butt, have a shower, and get ready to leave," gave me enough hope to ensure I was ready to be discharged the next day. This release was a testament to the power of determination, but mostly to the enduring strength that comes within a community willing and able to impart strength to you when you have none for yourself.

On November 19th, I went home, with 10 days of not eating having reduced my body mass by 25 pounds, just as it had the first time around.

-22-

The Days After

"You used to be much more ... 'muchier.' You've lost your muchness."

The Mad Hatter to Alice in Lewis Carroll, *Alice in Wonderland*

Like many things, recovery from surgery is sometimes as much in your head as it is in your body. Coming into the second surgery, there had been many unknowns about how quickly I would heal and what my quality of life would be. Since no one I'd spoken to had been able to give me any definitive information, I'd had to strike out on my own. Longer-term recovery was the same: in the words of my triathlon coach, it was, "Listen to your body, mate." Because surgery had inflicted major trauma to my body, the advice given me by Dr. Yaffe was, "Do not lift anything more than a few pounds for the next six weeks." I failed to follow that advice, and it caused me some problems down the road.

As the owner of a small business, I had to pick up where I'd left off when I'd entered the hospital. So, having exited the hospital on a Monday, I found myself in a client's office that Friday, having navigated my way downtown on the city bus and walked a couple of blocks through the patchy and semi-solid ice commonly found on the November sidewalks of Winnipeg. After an exhausting hour-long meeting, I walked four blocks to catch my bus home and, all the way, felt guilty because I chose to sit rather than give my seat up to the woman who got on a few stops after me (a choice made because I feared tearing my staples out by riding for half an hour with my full weight supported against the turns, stops, and lurches of the bus by a raised arm).

Later that day it snowed, and, fearing that my "good-for-some-things-only" children would not respond with enthusiasm to an admonition to shovel the driveway, I did it myself. Having completed the task, I fell onto the couch, exhausted.

As expected, day by day my strength returned. Before my surgery, a nurse had talked with me about expectations regarding mobility and the things I wanted to be able to do post surgery. Having queried me about whether or not my house had stairs and whether I'd need to be able to negotiate them on a day-to-day basis, she'd asked, "How far can you walk?" I think this was a diagnostic question designed to determine my level of fitness (at the time, I was 5'10" and weighed about 265 pounds) and to help set my expectations for mobility right after surgery. A little confused, I'd replied, "Well, 20, 30 kilometres." She'd laughed and checked some box on her survey.

The first Sunday after I was released from hospital, I walked two kilometres, deciding on that day I did not want to be fat any more. While it would take a couple of tries before I could make a lifestyle change significant enough to take my excess weight off permanently, that day I started a quest which would find me, in the fall of 2012, crossing the finish line in my first Ironman race.

Other things were working themselves out. While my small intestine did not work quite as effectively as my large one had, it was learning to adapt to being the king of my digestive system. At first I made many trips to the bathroom each day, but slowly, it was realizing it had to pick up the slack and started learning to do so, to some extent. As Chief Inspector Dryfuss, head of the French Sûreté, famously said, "Every day and in every way, I'm getting better and better."

Eye on the Horizon

"Never forget, that until the day that God deigns to reveal the future to man, all human wisdom is contained in these two words, - 'Wait and hope.' - Your friend, Edmund, Count of Monte Cristo." The eyes of both were fixed on the spot indicated by the sailor, and on the blue-line separating the sky from the Mediterranean Sea, they perceived a large white sail.

Alexandre Dumas, *The Count of Monte Cristo*

Physical recovery is a series of steps and decisions: some of them easy, some hard, some of them small, some large. It involves the choice to get up when you'd rather lie down. It's the choice to make lifestyle changes when the status quo is the easier path. Sometimes it involves trusting the advice of the experts, and sometimes it means trusting yourself.

Once my surgical therapy was complete, I had another hurdle to overcome, that of cancer follow-up. My first tumour had been classified as stage IA, which means a tumour confined to the surface of the intestine (accounting for the numeric value "I") with no lymph node involvement (accounting for the alpha value "A"). Thus, once the tumour and surrounding tissue with lymph nodes had been excised, the determination was that neither chemotherapy nor radiation therapy was required. As a result, I'd had no experience with oncologists, CancerCare, or chemotherapy in the years after my first cancer. My surgeon, Dr. Pfeifer, was only doctor I'd seen after surgery; he had conducted all the necessary follow-up and surveillance. Had he ever found anything of concern, he would have reported it to CancerCare, the provincial medical institution which oversees oncology cases.

The second experience would prove to be quite different, however. My second tumour was staged as a IIA malignancy, having begun to invade the inner wall of my intestine, although the good news was that none of the 41 lymph nodes they took out showed any sign of cancer. Nevertheless, with all tumours there is a risk that microscopic cancer cells might be present at the original site, even after the visible evidence has been removed. That risk increases as the depth to which the tumour has progressed in and through the initial organ grows. As a result, the follow-up regimen after surgery may involve a series of chemotherapy or radiation treatments, designed to kill off any cancer that might be present even though it won't show up on a scope, CT scan, or even under a pathologist's microscope. Soon after my surgery, while I'd still been in hospital, I'd received word that an oncologist had been assigned to me. The name bode well: it was Dr. Smith, the specialist our friend Marilyn had highly recommended.

Chemotherapy can be used in a variety of ways to treat malignant solid tumours such as the mass I had. It can be used to shrink inoperable tumours to reduce pain and extend life. It can also be used as neoadjuvant therapy, sometimes together with radiation therapy, to shrink tumours prior to surgery so as to make the surgery more effective. In a common treatment called adjuvant therapy, it is used post-operatively to target cancer cells that cannot be seen but are still suspected to be present. While I was recovering in hospital, I'd been told it was likely I'd be put through a course of adjuvant therapy because, despite the appearance that the cancer had all been removed through surgery, there was no way to be absolutely sure. So, post-surgery I awaited word about my upcoming meeting with Dr. Smith to talk about my specific treatment.

I met with Dr. Smith (not his real name) a few weeks after being released from the hospital. Over the next three months—although it certainly seemed longer—what should have been a story of pills, nausea, and hair loss turned instead into a quest for truth within the labyrinth of standard protocol and the bewildering resistance of a doctor assigned to help me through it.

My brother-in-law lives in the Caribbean, the product of personal ambition, skills, and the disproportionate number of Canadian banks in the area. I have stood there on the beach and watched the waves gently lap against the sand, with the strong sun and perhaps a cooling breeze on my face. I have set out on a boat, destined for some coral reef I could explore with my scuba gear and the help of a local guide. And from the moment I entered the watery depths, it was evident a completely different world existed under the surface I had just traversed: one which was quite a bit more interesting and, in some ways, more important than the one I exited into as I broke the ocean surface once again.

Sometimes, even from the surface, that undersea world can become evident. Sometimes it is a flash, a glint of light against something; other

times it is a fin breaking the surface; and sometimes it is the surfacing of
some great behemoth, the aquatic remnant of a bygone age.

My journey to full health, the one that started the moment surgery
was complete and continued as I went home to convalesce, should have
been just a trip around some craggy island—albeit a distant one—and
back again. High winds, sunburn, perhaps some squalls, rain, and
rough water, but nothing I could not manage. What actually happened,
however, was wholly unexpected. At first, a glint from under the surface,
a flash; but by the end, what had emerged from the water completely
subverted the planned journey and reoriented my way of thinking.

-24-

Surface Tension

"I am afraid," said [Watson], "that the facts are so obvious that you will find little credit to be gained out of this case."

"There is nothing more deceptive than an obvious fact," [Holmes] answered, laughing. "Besides, we may chance to hit upon some other obvious facts which may have been by no means obvious to Mr. Lestrade."

Arthur Conan Doyle, "The Bascombe Valley Mystery" in *The Adventures of Sherlock Holmes*

As I was engrossed in recovering from surgery, a parallel story was unfolding next to me. One that I occasionally intersected with, but which moved along largely without my effort or involvement. The story was that of my wife, Debra, and our friend, Rob James, who was living on Salt Spring Island, off the west coast of British Columbia. Rob is an epidemiologist by training and vocation, which means he is a statistics man with a deep interest in the status and trends of all things to do with diseases.

Rob is the kind of person you want around when you are trying to discover medical information in published articles (such as those found in the *New England Journal of Medicine* and *The Lancet*) but lack the vocabulary to understand the terminology and the mathematical skills to grasp all the implications of the statistics, especially the nuances. The bottom line is that Rob loves nothing better than to sit down with a journal article and cup of coffee and make sense out of the puzzle that is medical research and its reporting. He has alerts set up on medical web sites to email him when articles with key words for the subjects he is interested in are published. To this day, he continues to forward relevant material to us, so we can remain abreast of developments in understanding and treating Lynch syndrome.

While I was busy trying to figure out how my body, fresh from major surgery and missing a large organ, was supposed to function, Rob began to search out information, keeping an eagle eye out for the world centres of excellence in Lynch syndrome—those loci of research and repositories of knowledge that are so critical when dealing with a rare disease. Debra and he began to unearth and familiarize themselves with research pertaining to the genetic malady that had generated my two cancers.

In this way, what would otherwise have been one story—of my chemotherapy and visits to oncologists and CancerCare—became two intersecting stories. As with many tangled tales, one thread was straightforward and the other convoluted and complicated. Over time, the complex story under the sea began to subsume the story on the surface. Very few people experienced the undersea story firsthand, although more heard about its frustration and even desperation; it happened, in large part, without even my own full awareness. It was the story filled with investigation and research, knowledge and speculation, contradiction and fears. The obvious story on the surface would have progressed without incident, presumably, were it not for the hidden one raising its head occasionally, barely perceptible at first but culminating in such a splash and froth that the other could not help but simply sink into the depths. But, I am getting ahead of myself: should I have said, "Spoiler alert"?

As early as the date of my surgery, my background bookworms had been working. Rob had been diligently accessing cutting-edge research in the medical literature to find information about Lynch syndrome and its treatments. Whenever he found an article of interest, he'd email it to Debra and copy it to me, along with commentary about how relevant or compelling the article was and what the potential implications were. As a statistician, he had great insight into the meaning of the numbers associated with the results of the studies, and as the husband of a doctor, he had gleaned further medical expertise by osmosis. I generally skimmed the articles, but Debra poured over them, several varicoloured highlighters in hand, often struggling to understand all the terminology, the finer points of cell biochemistry, the statistical offerings, and research methodologies, but with dogged determination to fully grasp the implications and nuances of all the research.

Their research continued apace until one red-letter day in the middle of December, 2007, when we got an email from Rob that said, "Now THIS is interesting." It was an important study he'd found in the *New England Journal of Medicine*, penned right next door in Ontario by Drs. Robert Gryfe and Steven Gallinger. This article, published in

2000, asserted that tumours characterized as having high microsatellite instability (MSI-H), representing 90% of those produced by people with Lynch syndrome, were fundamentally different from regular, spontaneous tumours and needed to be recognized as a clinically distinct subtype. In 2003, these doctors again published in the same prestigious medical journal, presenting research which showed that in stage II and III MSI-H tumours, the use of adjuvant chemotherapy was, at best, ineffective and, at worst, lowered the five-year survival rate of patients. Moreover, Rob discovered that one of the authors, Dr. Gallinger, headed the Ontario Familial Colorectal Cancer Registry, an ongoing colorectal cancer research project and the largest of its kind in Canada. It was momentous to have discovered a world-class concentration of Lynch research and expertise so close to home, right in Canada and, in fact, in our neighbouring province.

In the meantime, I'd received notice in the mail telling me I'd be meeting with Dr. Smith on December 18th. Given what we'd been reading, we wondered whether he would be inclined to recommend chemotherapy, as would be quite possible with regular stage II colon cancer, or whether he'd be interested in discussing the differences in treatment for a Lynch tumour.

As would become their pattern, Rob and Debra conferred the night before my first appointment with Dr. Smith. They decided that the key piece of information to glean during the appointment, outside of Dr. Smith's recommendation regarding chemotherapy, was where the world centres of excellence for Lynch syndrome were, expecting that while he would certainly identify Dr. Gallinger's clinic and the Toronto researchers we had been reading, he would also cite other loci of Lynch-focused research. We wanted to ensure that we had not missed anything, and we wanted to engage in discussion with Dr. Smith over the findings of the Toronto Lynch researchers.

And so, on December 18th, 2007, Debra and I entered the clinic of Dr. Smith, looking forward to the reassurance of an illuminating conversation about Lynch syndrome cancers and the ins and outs of their treatment.

"Hello, Dennis. I'm Dr. Smith and will be treating you."

"Hello, Dr. Smith. What's the course of treatment?"

"I want to wait until your body heals sufficiently from the surgery, as well as for the holiday season to be over, so we can wait until January to start treatment. However, at that time, we'll start you on a regimen of adjuvant chemotherapy. While the stage of your tumour is relatively low, at IIA, your young age is an important high-risk factor to consider. You can choose the traditional method of delivery for the chemotherapy, through a port installed in your body which will be hooked up to the drugs on regular visits to the hospital. Alternatively, you have the option of a more recent and, for most people, more convenient form of chemotherapy, Xeloda, which is administered orally."

"The oral chemotherapy sounds preferable to me. What are the side effects of the chemotherapy? Will I lose my hair?"

"Many people experience few to no side effects with this chemotherapy. You might experience some hair loss, but that is by no means guaranteed. You may also experience some tingling or numbing of your hands and feet—sometimes called *hand–foot*—as well as some stomach upset, especially with certain kinds of food. The oral treatment has a lot of advantages, primarily because you do not need an IV port, and also because you can take it at home rather than coming in here for treatment."

"How long will I have to do chemo?"

"You'll do eight rounds for now. This means taking pills for two weeks, followed by a week of recovery. You'll repeat that three-week cycle eight times, for a total of six months."

"Okay."

"Here is your prescription. You'll start taking the pills during the first week of January—let's say January 3rd—and I'll meet with you at the end of that first round to talk about how the chemo went. My assistant will be in touch with you to schedule your appointments. Do you have any questions?"

"Yes, we have a few. What can you tell me about where the world centres of excellence are for Lynch syndrome?"

He shook his head. "There aren't any."

Taken aback and referring to the list of questions in her hand, Debra stammered, "Well, we have some questions here we hoped you'd address. They're based on Dr. Gallinger's research on chemotherapy for MSI-H tumours, which Lynch syndrome usually produces."

Debra wanted to find out about more about the preliminary research we'd done, but Dr. Smith, while aware of Dr. Gallinger's work, said the research done to date on microsatellite instability in tumours had no clinical relevance. He also clarified that my tumour being the result of Lynch syndrome was not germane to his treatment considerations; he was approaching my case just as he would a sporadic, or standard, case of colorectal cancer.

Debra and I left the office, my wife alarmed and discouraged by what she'd heard, as well as what she'd not heard—answers to the questions we had come with. For my part, I was not yet well versed or really invested in the information that Debra, Rob, and Marilyn were so critically assessing. For the time being, I was content to move forward with Dr. Smith's plan to take pills containing a drug called capecitabine, sold as Xeloda.

The standard in-clinic treatment for colorectal cancer is an intravenous drug called 5-Fluorouracil (5-FU). In the adjuvant therapy I was getting for stage II—more of a precautionary treatment given when there's a chance of cancer being in the body but no clinical evidence that it's there—capecitabine is a frequently favoured alternative. When it is ingested and absorbed by the body, its chemical formulation changes into 5-FU once it reaches the cancerous cells. For many people, the side effects are less severe than with the IV treatments, so it seemed that my flowing mane of blonde hair (at least what remained after some age-related erosion) would be safe from the ravages of chemotherapy.

I would follow a regimen of two weeks on and then one week off. This would allow the chemicals to build to their maximum toxicity (towards the cancer, but which the rest of my body had to be able to withstand). My body would then get a break while it tried to recover from the damages. I would repeat this three-week process eight times and then get a CT scan to see if there was any evidence of tumour growth at the site of the surgery.

This plan continued to cause more than a bit of a stir in our household, however. In great consternation over the impending start of a chemotherapy she feared might harm more than help me—indeed perhaps end my life—Debra explained to Rob and Marilyn that Dr. Smith thought the research regarding the insensitivity of MSI-H tumours to chemotherapy was not clinically relevant.

"Oh, but it is relevant," said Marilyn. "It is." She was as confused and concerned over the lack of traction our concerns had had with Dr. Smith as Debra was.

On December 20th, Debra took the first step towards securing a second opinion. She emailed Dr. Steven Gallinger, presenting my situation, including many details from the surgery pathology report she'd procured a copy of, explaining our awareness of his team's research and its apparent implications for my care, and indicating my oncologist's resolve to treat me as a standard colorectal cancer patient rather than as a Lynch-specific case. She clicked "Send" with high hopes of a favourable response.

A few days later, she got a brief reply from Dr. Gallinger, explaining that he was reluctant to make recommendations by email and that he could not elaborate beyond what we had already gleaned from the research we'd found. However, he did recommend that we get the tumour tested to see if it was MSI-H.

The team of three decided to get busy. First, they would continue to gather more research, prepare a bibliography, and present their questions and concerns to Dr. Smith in a concise but thorough email: the next office appointment was a long month away. They had their work cut out for them. In the days that followed, when they weren't feverishly emailing back and forth, the team were phoning.

Next, given Dr. Gallinger's recommendation for testing and the critical role of MSI status in chemotherapy treatment, Debra called Dr. Smith's office to ask whether my tumour tissue could be tested to discover its level of microsatellite instability. At the same time, she asked whether Dr. Smith would give me a referral to Dr. Gallinger. Debra was not able to speak directly with Dr. Smith, but his assistant conferred with him on our behalf and advised Debra that the local lab would not be able to test my tumour for its MSI status, nor would Dr. Smith be referring me to Dr. Gallinger.

In contrast to the frenetic activity of my research team, my own disposition was to follow inertia. Set me on a path, and I'll put my heart and soul into it until something interrupts my trajectory. And so, content to follow Dr. Smith's recommendation, I filled my first prescription for Xeloda. On January 3rd, 2008, I started taking one pill three times a day.

You never really understand the cost of health care until you have to shell out of your pocket for things. Having lived in Canada my entire life, I am used to going to the doctor when I am sick, or showing up at the hospital when I need urgent treatment for sprains, strains, and broken limbs, and not worrying about anything beyond my health card, which I carry around regularly, much as I do my driver license. However, one thing Canada has not fully implemented is a universal drug program; that is, some way to ensure that critical medications are made available to all, whether you can afford them or not. Up until this point, I'd had experience with purchasing Aspirin and the occasional prescription for antibiotics; I had even seen some high-priced medications for Debra's increasing number of migraines. But that was it. So even though I'd heard stories of prescription drugs bankrupting people because of their high cost, I was completely unprepared for the price of chemotherapy. When Debra brought home my first week of pills, I took the container, glanced at the cost, and set it aside. Then, like a cartoon character who has just realized he has run off the edge of a cliff but not yet begun to fall, I shook my head and took another look. With naïve incredulity, I asked, "Is that $1000 for the whole month?"

"No, just two weeks."

I sat for a few seconds, just staring at the cost of the drugs on the bottle and doing the math in my head. Realizing what I was doing, Debra reassured me, "Don't worry. We only had to meet our PharmaCare deductible, so much of the cost was covered. We won't have to pay for any more—at least until April when the year rolls over."

"PharmaCare?"

"Yes, the provincial drug program!"

Debra was surprised I didn't know about the program, typical of all Canadian provinces, although the details can vary among jurisdictions.

Ironically, were I to have gone to the CancerCare clinic in the hospital to get chemotherapy, I would have had to pay nothing out of pocket because virtually all hospital treatment is fully covered by the public health care system. Due to this anomaly, some patients choose IV chemotherapy simply out of concern over the high cost of their deductible for the oral prescription drugs (not all deductibles are equal, nor are all drugs even covered by all provinces). The real irony is that such budget-conscious choices end up costing the government exponentially more. All hospital treatment is very costly, so even if the government were to absorb the full cost of oral chemotherapy with no deductible to the patient, it would still save vast amounts of public funds. It really is a stunning example of a lose–lose situation. All this a product of the chaotic implementation and management of health care in Canada. Sigh, if only I were the benevolent dictator, the philosopher-king of Canada, some people would have some '*splainin'* to do.

So, I took my drugs and lived my life. I travelled out of town for work (something I could do only because I was taking oral chemo) and experienced what I think was my first chemo-related side effect: burning when I went to the bathroom. Later on, I would be told by a CancerCare nurse that it was probably due to spicy foods combined with a diet high in tomato-based foods such as BBQ sauce.

Debra worried about the powerful drugs I had begun to ingest. Besides the evidence of inefficacy and even potential harm in the *New England Journal of Medicine* study and elsewhere, she was also contemplating the idea that a body already highly vulnerable to cancer didn't need further weakening by having to deal with toxic chemicals coursing through it.

Early into January, Rob and Debra had amassed a library of scholarly articles from the databases they had scoured. They were pursuing the course of inquiry suggested by the initial papers they'd located prior to our first meeting with Dr. Smith, which proposed that my body produced a fundamentally different type of tumour than sporadic or standard colorectal cancer and that, as a result, the Lynch cancer needed to be treated differently. Rob and Debra hunted down all the information they could find; the preponderance of evidence supporting that proposition was compelling, while the scholarly voices opposing it were fewer and weaker. It was time to email Dr. Smith. They crafted a careful, succinct presentation of the content and its implications for my case.

By this time, my team harboured grave misgivings about my taking chemotherapy. Debra was particularly concerned that the MSI status of my tumour be confirmed, so she also phoned the Mayo clinic in Rochester, New York, to see if the testing could be done there. The process was not straightforward, however, and cost was a consideration.

Day by day, perhaps hour by hour, Debra waited for a reply from Dr. Smith, checking the email inbox frequently, hoping to get some sort of feedback and engagement on what all this research meant in terms of my treatment. A follow-up email went out into the abyss of cyberspace, but nary a word was heard in response. To Debra, the silence was profoundly upsetting. She felt the pressure of the increasing length of time that I was taking chemo. Even worse, she felt at sea with no oncological expert at the helm of our little bateau in the storm waters: answers seemed no closer now than they had been at the outset.

On January 13th, 2008, I awoke in the morning, looked to the bottle of pills on my bedside table, and decided that I'd had enough. I considered the two courses of action that lay ahead of me: taking the pills and finishing the course of treatment that Dr. Smith had set out or admitting that the weight of evidence was sufficient to persuade me that I should be on a different road altogether. I decided on the latter. It was not a decision I took lightly, nor did I make it because I thought chemotherapy was, in its essence, a poor choice for cancer treatment. Rather, based on the weight of scientific evidence, I decided that it was not right for me. So the pill bottle remained on my bedside table, whence it would eventually move into a drawer.

I was done. I had taken one and a half weeks of chemotherapy, and I was done with that treatment. It would be a couple of days before I told Debra. I was concerned that she would judge my decision, made without the blessing of an oncologist, as rash. As expected, when I did tell her, she did not feel unmixed relief; rather, she felt heightened pressure to gain Dr. Smith's ear on the matter of Lynch considerations. Either that or the specific engagement of Dr. Gallinger's team.

On January 17th, I had my first oncological appointment since starting chemotherapy. Debra and I arrived at the clinic, once again armed with a folder full of articles and an even longer list of questions for Dr. Smith, questions fully vetted with Rob and Marilyn and prepped down to the lingo with which we would present them. This time, I was a fully vested partner in the exercise. We saw this appointment as our last effort to get Dr. Smith to view me as a Lynch patient with cancer rather than as a cancer patient with Lynch syndrome.

"Hi Dennis! How is it going?"

"Well, chemo has not really been a problem. But I have some serious misgivings about continuing. The articles we are finding and have been emailing to you really seem to indicate this is not a good idea for me."

He conducted a brief examination, tapping my back. I breathed in and out a few times.

He sat down and pulled out his pad and began to write me a prescription for the next course of Xeloda.

"But what about the research regarding MSI and adjuvant chemotherapy in Lynch patients?"

"Yes, I reviewed those. The research is preliminary and not clinically relevant."

"But it seems to be relevant," Debra interjected. "The study about MSI seems to speak directly to Dennis' situation."

"No, it is really not applicable to this situation."

"Is it possible to speak to Dr. Gallinger in Toronto?" she pressed. "Could we phone him? Maybe he will be able to provide some insight into the clinical implications of his study."

"Perhaps we could, but what would be the point?"

"Well, the research points to the value of knowing if the tumour was MSI-high. Can we get the tissue tested?"

"No, we do not do that here."

"Can we get that done somewhere else?"

"The provincial government would never pay for that." He paused.

"Dennis, if you go off chemo, you can't just start again later. You have to commit now to doing this, and then follow through."

I nodded my understanding.

"Is that all?"

I look at Dr. Smith, dismayed and perplexed as to how to proceed.

"It appears to me that you are not committed to this course of treatment," he said. "I cannot have you going on and off chemotherapy. As a result, I'm not going to prescribe any more Xeloda to you." He tore off the prescription he was writing, crumpled it, and put it in his pocket.

"I think what we'll do is start the surveillance now, and I will see you in three months for your next follow-up."

We said our goodbyes, and Dr. Smith left the examining room. We collected our things, just as bewildered as we'd been at the end of our previous visit, but more discouraged. Despite his lack of response to our well-documented emails, we had gone in with a last-ditch hope that Dr. Smith would engage with us as relatively informed patients and weigh in on our specific questions and earnest concerns. For my part, I'd held out hope right to the end of the appointment for a conclusion that recognized the probable validity of my concerns and a shared recognition that chemo was not the right course of treatment for me.

While neither Debra nor I could be wholly surprised that our hopes hadn't materialized, neither were we prepared for Dr. Smith's ultimatum on continuing chemo without interruption or foregoing it altogether. Debra, already struggling with my abrupt halt of treatment, found this particularly unnerving. As we drove home, I could tell she was terrified that we might have to continue navigating these dark waters of the unknown without any oncologist on board.

I recall a phone conversation Debra had with Rob later that evening.

"Did he even read the articles?"

"We're not sure. It seemed he might have, but it wasn't clear. He just kept saying it wasn't clinically relevant. Then he said that Dennis couldn't restart chemo if he stopped. And that he couldn't continue chemo because he was too uncommitted."

"What about a consult with Dr. Gallinger?"

"He said something like, 'What's the point?'"

"Wow. Okay, let's figure out what we can do."

-25-

Connections

... that best portion of a good man's life;
His little, nameless unremembered acts
Of kindness and of love.

William Wordsworth, "Lines Written a Few Miles
Above Tintern Abby" in *Lyrical Ballads*

As the undersea activity continued, it had begun breaking the surface of my story more often, with increasing vigour and fury. Now, I was able to discern what the nature of the monster in the depths was: my Lynch syndrome. As I looked back over the previous month—a period of intense research, burning questions, and long discussion of treatment plans—I saw a consistent theme: a lack of fundamental acknowledgement that my Lynch syndrome had anything to do with the treatment of my cancer.

Debra and Rob were convinced it was only when we could speak with someone who saw both the cancer and the genetics that we would get real answers to our questions. Having experienced what they described through clenched teeth as *obstructionism*, Debra and Rob decided it was time to take matters into our own hands. The key was to connect with the clinic of Dr. Steven Gallinger. But how do you get a world-renowned research physician to take your call? Well, you begin with a world-renowned research scientist you happen to be related to.

The day after my second appointment with Dr. Smith, following another evening of intense discussion with Rob, we decided to reach out to the one person we thought was best able to understand our questions in light of the science and, at the same time, also able to put us in touch with Dr. Gallinger and his colleagues: Debra's mother's cousin, Canada Research Chair of Stem Cell Biology, Dr. John Dick of Toronto. "They're probably lunch buddies," quipped Rob.

Dr. Dick's early research into cancer stem cells revolutionized leukaemia therapy and the understanding of how blood cancers

generate and progress. His further research into the role of stem cells
in solid tumours was equally groundbreaking, and his lab continues
to make seminal contributions to the understanding of cancer and its
treatments. In 2004, Dr. Dick became a Fellow of the Royal Society of
Canada. In the summer of 2014—after years of careful vetting of his
credentials subsequent to his nomination—he was inducted as a Fellow
of the Royal Society, the oldest society dedicated to the advancement
of science, begun in 1660 and including Sir Isaac Newton, Charles
Darwin, and other luminaries. With his hallmark humility, John began
the email he reluctantly sent out to his relatives with these words: "This
is just a short note to say that I recently got some interesting news. Of
course it goes against my upbringing of 'guarding against pride' to make
too big a deal of this, but I knew you would want to know." He finishes,
"Still bending my head around this remarkable recognition. I can hear
Dad's voice in my ear saying, 'How can someone from that small farm
in Culross do that?'" So, not only is John a pre-eminent scientist, he is
a kindly, down-to-earth man who remembers his roots and who values
others, especially family.

On Saturday, January 19th, 2008, Debra began making local calls
in Winnipeg in an attempt to find contact information for John. After
getting a phone number where she could reach him at home, she dialled
with heightened anticipation but was disappointed to reach only his
voice mail.

"Hi, John. This is Debra Maione, your cousin Eleonore's
daughter. I'm hoping you can give me a call. My husband Dennis
has a rare kind of colorectal cancer, HNPCC, or Lynch syndrome,
and we are experiencing some trouble getting expert advice on the
recommendation he was given regarding chemotherapy. I hope you'll be
able to give me a call. Thanks."

Throughout that long evening we waited for a return call, but it
never came.

The next morning, after we'd been up for an hour, the phone rang.
Debra answered, and I saw her excitement: it was John Dick. In their
brief conversation, he apologized for taking so long to return her call.
He and his wife were in the airport on their way to Hong Kong, where
he was to address a conference. However, he suggested that he could
contact some people in Toronto who might be able to help us, including
a friend of his, a surgeon who specialized in Lynch syndrome, Dr.
Steven Gallinger.

Debra was nothing less than elated upon getting off the phone.

This seemed to be the break we had been looking for—the prospect of support that would lead to answers to our questions. She quickly typed up an email to John. Thanking him for calling, she explained in some detail the history of my situation to date, especially the rigours of the past month and our frustration in trying to get my Lynch syndrome recognized when it came to determining my treatment regime. It was 10:30 a.m. on Sunday, January 20th, 2008.

A flurry of emails quickly ensued. The sheer volume of activity that transpired in such a short period was a tribute not just to the stature of Dr. Dick, but also to his genuine care for others and to that same spirit in the people surrounding him. We were interacting with people whose appreciation of both the uniqueness and gravity of our situation made that remarkable level of progress possible.

At 11:15 a.m., Dr. Dick emailed his post-doctoral fellow, Dr. Catherine O'Brien, requesting her assistance in getting us a second opinion in Toronto. (Dr. O'Brien was herself a surgical oncologist with specialized interest in colorectal cancer.) In the coming days, she would take on the pivotal role of coordinating our interactions with the Lynch specialists in Toronto, as well as provide support and an understanding ear to Debra as she tried to find a way forward in this territory never before navigated.

At 5:57 p.m., Dr. O'Brien emailed Dr. Gallinger, explaining our situation but misinterpreting our request as our desiring a second opinion in Winnipeg.

At 8:48 a.m. on Monday, January 21st, Dr. Gallinger replied to Dr. O'Brien, indicating, much as he had to Debra when she'd contacted him in December, that it was hard to make recommendations without seeing me. In an ironic turn, he suggested that we try Dr. Smith in Winnipeg as a specialist who might be able to assist us in our predicament.

At 10:09 a.m., Dr. O'Brien emailed Debra to let her know what Dr. Gallinger had said. Moreover, having realized our original request was for a consultation in Toronto, she added that she would ask Dr. Gallinger to try to arrange a consultation with one of the medical oncologists he worked with.

Thrilled, Debra and I carefully crafted a tactful reply, explaining we had already consulted with Dr. Smith but had not found an audience for our questions and would therefore would be very grateful to go to Toronto. We also indicated that, should a referral be necessary, it would come from Dr. Yaffe.

At 6:07 p m , we received positive confirmation of our goal: we would be able to go to Toronto for a consultation with Drs. Steven Gallinger, surgical oncologist, and Malcolm Moore, medical oncologist, the latter being head of the Department of Medical Oncology and Haematology at Princess Margaret Hospital in Toronto. All that was left was for the logistics to be worked out once a date had been set for the Toronto consult. We were elated, on the cusp of appointments with two doctors in Canada who were arguably among the world's top experts in Lynch syndrome.

There were high-fives and the requisite call to Rob and Marilyn to tell them the good news. There would still be travail to come, but we seemed to be well on our way to the solution we required. The great monster from the deep had finally breached, and my voyage on the once deceptively calm surface had come to an end. I was no longer a cancer patient who had Lynch syndrome; I was a Lynch patient with cancer. This change of perspective, which I now realize was all I really wanted from Dr. Smith, would change the way I approached my disease and doctors henceforth.

By noon on January 22nd, we had confirmation from Dr. Moore's clinic that he would see me for a consultation and render a second opinion on the chemotherapeutic treatment of my cancer. In all, it had taken a little over 48 hours to connect with Canada's centre of Lynch syndrome excellence and get confirmation that the experts there would see me.

Now, in a country with socialized medicine, the invitation to come for a consultation is not sufficient to compel your home province, responsible for your medical treatment, to pay for services that you travel to another jurisdiction to receive. For that, you need to start with a referral from a specialist who is currently treating you. Given that Dr. Smith had declared his perspective that the Lynch research was irrelevant to my situation, it was back to Dr. Yaffe to rescue me once again.

I approached him with some trepidation, being a little concerned that he might take offence at being asked to refer me to another doctor for an expert opinion on my treatment: treatment that he was actively involved in, if only from a follow-up perspective. Furthermore, I had no idea how much consultation he might have had with Dr. Smith and whether that would come into play. That concern was to prove groundless, however; true to form, Dr. Yaffe, was more than happy to give me a referral to both Dr. Gallinger's and Dr. Moore's clinics.

The final hurdle was to get approval from the provincial government for the consultation and my travel expenses. By the beginning of February, Dr. Moore's clinic had phoned a couple of times to find out when I would be coming, first scheduling me and then rescheduling my appointment to a later date while we continued to await word.

Having worked for the provincial government for quite a while before we were married, Debra knew how slow the bureaucratic processes could be. And she was painfully conscious of the passage of time, which worried her should my tumour test as MSI-low after all, or should the doctors in Toronto decide for some other reason that chemo was indeed best for me. Moreover, she was concerned not only about a potentially long delay but also that the government's ruling might not be in our favour, so that we would be left struggling to fund the trip and consultation on our own when our finances were already stressed.

Rather than simply wait, Debra tried to help move things along, deciding to call the office of Theresa Oswald, then Minister of Health for Manitoba. While she never did speak to the Minister herself, she got reasonably close, speaking with an aide who wielded some influence—influence which was possibly an effective part of the process that saw our application looked at and approved at the first available opportunity. Years later, I was to share the podium with the same Minister at the announcement of a new cancer genetics research facility to be constructed; Ms. Oswald complimented me highly on my speech, but I never got the opportunity to tell her about the role that her department, and perhaps her assistant, had played in my journey.

The coveted approval to travel came through several days later. It was February 13th, 2008. We booked our flights to Toronto, arranging to stay with friends while we were there. And for the first time in months, we relaxed and breathed in the air of promise.

Recalling that period of December 2007 through February 2008, Debra recently told me how difficult she'd found it, constantly feeling scared for me. "First, I struggled so hard to find out what the correct course of action was, yet felt as though we were always hitting a brick wall. And you were resistant to any thought that Dr. Smith might be wrong or that chemo might not be right for you. I feared chemo might kill you—if not directly, then perhaps by crippling your body's ability to fight future cancers. Then, out of the blue, you suddenly invested yourself in the research Rob and I had found and stopped chemo, just like that! While there was relief in that, there was also fear: what if I'd been the catalyst for behaviour that ended up costing you your life? Without an oncologist at the helm of all that research, I felt virtually as much angst after your decision as I had before."

So the Toronto trip was critical for Debra, but I am built differently. Had it not worked out, I would have been content with my decision. That is the way I tend to see life: you look at your options and choose. Once the decision has been made, you never look back and wonder whether it was the right one, because it was the one you made, and nothing—never mind mere wondering or second-guessing—can change the past.

Be that as it may, Toronto was very important in our lives, both then and in years to come. And our trip in February, 2008 was to prove memorable on a number of levels. We enjoyed the warm hospitality of Ellen, Debra's longtime friend from undergraduate days, and her husband, Loftus, with whom we shared rich camaraderie over wine and a meal on the day of our arrival.

The next evening, February 19th, Debra and I found ourselves in Hugh's Room, a small club in Toronto, for a concert Rob had highly recommended and which we attended out of deference to him. It proved to be yet another inestimable gift from our west coast friend. We were profoundly moved as we listened to a phenomenal array of artists play both with and for the stellar fiddler, Oliver Schroer. The concert was a tribute to him as well as a fund-raiser: only a few months earlier, Oliver had been diagnosed with leukaemia. He was in the midst of chemotherapy and awaiting a bone-marrow transplant. A highly influential musician, Oliver was so beloved that a large group of young fiddlers had flown in from B.C. to surprise him that evening. The atmosphere filled with love and seeming magic as they suddenly poured into the room, fiddling his distinctive music, wearing glowing lights, and wheeling and swirling around all the tables. Oliver smiled broadly as he played with them. CBC's Shelagh Rogers was the emcee for the evening, and Canada's national broadcasting station was recording the feast of music.

While Oliver appeared to be energetic and in good health during his performances, I noticed, as the concert went on, something hanging out of the top of his V-necked shirt: the port, implanted in his chest some months earlier, for the convenient delivery of his chemotherapy. To this day, listening to his CDs takes me back to that poignant evening and to the array of emotions we experienced those few days we spent in Toronto. Despite the sense of a hallowed evening and the hope and inspiration which the music and fellowship evoked in all who attended, Oliver Schroer was never to receive that bone-marrow transplant: just a few months later, in June of 2008, he died from his cancer. His music was one of the many legacies that he left behind from his too-short excursion in this life.

On Wednesday, February 20th, I found myself where I could not have imagined being just over a month earlier: in an examining room with Drs. Steven Gallinger and Malcolm Moore, discussing my situation with them. It is still hard to believe that we actually got that audience. It seems a lot like getting the opportunity to sit down with Stephen Hawking to talk about black holes. But we were nothing if not persistent, and, in the end, we were able to sit down with the very best.

The good doctors had seen my medical charts which had been forwarded by Dr. Yaffe, and the consultation was brief and to the point.

"Has the tumour been tested for MSI?"

"No. Dr. Smith said we could not get that done."

"Well, we could do it here, but I suppose the question is moot as your Lynch status has been confirmed, and, as a result, it is almost guaranteed that your tumour is MSI-high."

"What does that mean to me regarding adjuvant chemo?"

Dr. Gallinger looked to Dr. Moore, who said, "Well, nobody likes to tell anyone with cancer not to take chemo, in case there is a bad end, and one fears the advice was bad. However, if it were I, I wouldn't take it."

And that was it, as far as the consult was concerned. It was as simple as that: "I wouldn't take it."

The burning question that we'd brought had been answered, and I was definitely not going to continue with chemotherapy. We thanked them fervently and asked to have their recommendation forwarded to Dr. Yaffe for my files. They requested my permission to requisition a sample of my tumour tissue to ensure it was tested for MSI and the data entered into their research files.

Debra and I spent the afternoon with Spring Holter, a genetic counsellor and integral part of the Familial Gastrointestinal Cancer Registry, also under Dr. Gallinger's purview. She ran me through a gamut of questions about my own medical history and those of my relatives. Debra and I pulled out reams of paper along with a large scroll documenting my family tree and its cancer cases. Of course, we talked a lot about our children, the concerns we had regarding their genetic status, and the implications of their carrying the same mutation as I did.

Debra and I heartily enjoyed interacting with Spring, who brought her delightful and sparkling personality to a difficult job. She told us we were the most informed genetics patients she'd ever had—a function, I suppose, of the need we'd had to break our own trail for this journey.

During our conversation, I remarked to Spring that one of the best things about having had my whole colon removed recently was that I could stop having colonoscopies and their attendant oral gastrointestinal lavages, replacing them with sigmoidoscopies, which required only enemas to clean me out.

Spring responded, "I have never heard anyone celebrate enemas before!" I guess she just does not go to the right parties.

We left Princess Margaret Hospital that day fully satisfied and buoyed by an overwhelming sense of relief, knowing that our line of inquiry and my resultant decision had been correct, and also knowing that we had support from clinicians who had it made it a significant part of their life's work to understand the cancers resulting from my genetic condition. A clinical door which had been firmly closed to us had now swung wide and was being held open by some of the world's best minds on the subject. We felt as though we'd established a lifeline for our family.

It was on that day that I first felt part of a community that was like me. Since discovering that I have Lynch syndrome and my cancers are the result of a defective gene, I have felt very much alone in my experience. While the cancer journey itself is tragically all too common, and while standard colorectal cancer is also very common, tumours resulting from Lynch syndrome are rare. As a result, I've often felt myself to be an anomaly in the community of cancer survivors: genetics-related issues, an old man's cancer at a young age, no prolonged chemotherapy, and relatively few ill effects either before or after. I sometimes feel as though I never had "real" cancer because my journey has not been filled with the degree of pain, loss, and suffering that so many others have experienced.

The second and most profound time that I experienced this sense of being part of a community was two and a half years later at a day-long seminar held in Vancouver, B.C., where I sat in a room with a host of people who also had Lynch syndrome and who, I could say, were "just like me." Some were in the midst of cancer, others had their cancers behind them, and some were so-called *previvors*, facing the statistical likelihood of getting cancer at some point in their future. On that occasion, I got to chat with a young man who was in the same situation

I'd been in as a newlywed 15 years earlier, recently diagnosed with cancer that had struck like a lightning bolt. It was deeply satisfying to be able to sit down with this young man, to tell him that he was not alone, to assure him there were others who had experienced the same things he was going through, and to tell him it was going to be okay.

The next couple of months after returning from Toronto went by fairly uneventfully. I had my first follow-up appointment with Dr. Smith in April. By that point, I had begun running, training quite a bit in preparation for my first half-marathon—all part of the lifestyle changes I was making. At that visit to the oncologist, I commented I was finding blood in my shorts after I ran, an observation that served to accelerate the schedule for my next scope, bumping it up to June. Thankfully, the colonoscopy showed everything was clear: it is likely the blood came from chafing on my legs rather than discharge from my digestive system.

In November of that year, I had my first post-surgery CT scan, and a week later, on the 25th, another follow-up appointment with Dr. Smith. The scan had revealed what he described as a "borderline node;" that is, a lymph node that seemed to be irritated but not indicative of any specific problems. I was concerned, but my fear was allayed by his confidence that it was probably nothing and his assurance that another CT scan would be done in a year to look for change.

Clean scopes followed in December of 2008 and June and December of 2009, a period punctuated by visits with Dr. Smith every three months. There was no sign of cancer—and that was not for a lack of looking. My final CT scan was on October 8th, 2009, which proved to be clean as well. At that point, the regular CT scans ceased because the risk of deleterious effects from the radiation began to outweigh the diagnostic benefits. I continued to see Dr. Smith every three months for another year, after which my visits were cut back to every six months and, eventually, to once a year.

By 2010, Lynch syndrome and its cancer had ceased to be a monster in the dark, rather having become a path I had to tread, rough at times, but one where I could recognize and negotiate the pitfalls. I had an established course of yearly sigmoidoscopy plus gastroscopy (the latter a surveillance of my upper-intestinal tract added in response to further Lynch risks) via Dr. Yaffe, and I continued to see Dr. Smith yearly for blood work and the five-minute tap, tap, tap, "breathe in, breathe out" examination that is my oncological follow-up.

Rob continued to track developments in medical research about

Lynch syndrome and colorectal cancer, and he was alerted to a study in the December, 2009 issue of *The Lancet*, published by John Burn, a geneticist in the United Kingdom who was soon to become Sir John Burn in recognition of his significant contribution to medical research. The study investigated the efficacy of Aspirin as an antineoplastic therapy for colon tumours in people with Lynch syndrome. To the layperson, what the study showed was promising results in the prevention of colon cancer through daily ingestion of ASA (acetyl-salicylic acid, the active ingredient in Aspirin). A significant reduction in the occurrence of colon cancer was shown in people who took daily doses of 600 mg, the rough equivalent of two standard-sized tablets. So, at my next appointment, on January 7th, 2010, two months after the second-year anniversary of my surgery, I approached Dr. Smith with this research to ask his opinion on what I should do.

"Hi, Dennis. How are you?"

"I'm well, thanks," I said as he tapped my back and listened to my breathing. "Hey, I found this research out of the UK talking about the use of Aspirin to help prevent colon cancer in Lynch syndrome. How do you think that could work for me?"

"The research is preliminary; I would not take any stock in it."

"Do you think that it can hurt to take it? Or that a lower dose than in the study might still help?"

"I will not make any recommendations based on research that is this preliminary."

That was it. Once more, I felt dismissed. I started taking therapeutic Aspirin anyway—one "baby" Aspirin per day—figuring that Burn's large study was compelling enough to warrant doing so. I have an uncomfortably high likelihood of future cancer to contend with, even with my colon virtually gone. Moreover, there are so many people in the general population taking small daily doses for heart problems that I was willing to join them. While the therapy is not without risk of gastrointestinal bleeds, the risk level is small enough that I was willing to undertake it once I got Dr. Kyeremateng to clear my H-Pylori levels. Certainly, I thought, Aspirin could not be nearly as harmful as the chemotherapy I was supposed to have taken post-surgery.

-26-

Life in the Gap

Gentle reader, may you never feel what I then felt! May your eyes never shed such stormy, scalding, heart-wrung tears as poured from mine. May you never appeal to Heaven in prayers so hopeless and so agonised as in that hour left my lips; for never may you, like me, dread to be the instrument of evil to what you wholly love.

Charlotte Brontë, *Jane Eyre*

So, that is the end of the middle of my story. Most of my story has not been written yet, I suppose. I am middle-aged, and I hope that I have 30–35 good years left. These days, I actually think about genetics more than I do cancer, primarily because cancer is a symptom, for me. A symptom of something much more insidious, the tendency of my body to let cancer start and to grow quickly; potentially, it could grab me again one day, despite the best efforts of my doctors.

We have had all of our kids tested for the mutation. According to standard protocols, children should start getting scoped 10 years before the earliest onset of a Lynch cancer in their direct family line. For our kids, that would have meant starting with colonoscopies at age 17. However, if testing could show they did not have my mutation, they could avoid the demanding surveillance regime—never the mind the joy of discovering they had been excluded from the Lynch club. Not wanting to put them through the ordeal of colonoscopies unnecessarily, we had them all tested, with their informed consent, between ages 15 and 18. I have had a lot of hard days with my kids (geniuses are hard to live with sometimes), but certainly one of the most difficult ever was the day my middle child, our eldest son, Alex, was told he had gotten the Lynch gene from me. I wept when I apologized for the trauma it was going to cause him—not that it was my fault, but parental guilt is not always logical, nor is its grip to be underestimated.

I can remember sitting and having coffee with Debra, some years earlier, as we'd talked about the implications of any of our kids having the gene. Knowing that some doctors were recommending prophylactic hysterectomies for women who had the Lynch gene once they completed their families, I'd teared up as I said to her, "And now, I am in the position of hoping that if one of our kids has this mutation, it will be one of the boys." What guilt comes with even the involuntary consideration of that choice, never mind assenting to it and knowing that if the choice were actually mine to make—rather than being the result of the law of large numbers—that is what I would do.

I love my kids, none more than the others (although the desire to throw them off a tall building comes and goes with the vagaries of each child and the circumstances they put me into). But I have always had the most tempestuous relationship with my son Alex, as well as the most compassion for him. He and I are very alike and, as a result, have the most strained relationship in the household. He is strong-willed and highly intelligent (much smarter than I am), but he is also fragile and insecure. Sometimes I understand him, and other times I feel profoundly disconnected from the way he sees the world. I have no idea what Lynch syndrome will mean for him, but at least he has a significant advantage over me. Between yearly scopes and daily Aspirin therapy, it is likely that any polyps that form will be detected and removed before they ever reach the cancerous stage, despite the presence of the mutated gene in him. The bonus of all this is that he and I share a bond I have with no one else. And I have been where he is going as far as surveillance is concerned, and even cancer and surgery, should these ever befall him. He is his own man, but, once a year, at least for the time being, we get to share a room in the *Not for Admitting* ward at the St. Boniface Hospital as we await our scopes. Nothing like a bit of a cleanse, fast, and scope outing to bring a father and son closer together.

When All You Have Is a Hammer

When you hear hoof beats, think horses, not zebras.

Author Unknown (though he'd obviously not been on safari in Africa)

Abraham Maslow once wrote, "I suppose it is tempting, if the only tool you have is a hammer, to treat everything as if it were a nail." And to that I reply, "When you have a cancer gene in your family, intestinal distress always looks like cancer." At least, that is the way it seemed in the fall of 2012 when my son, Noah, ended up in the hospital with pain in his abdomen.

He has always had issues with his gut, ongoing distress that comes and goes. But, on that October morning, the pain seemed extraordinarily bad—so much so that, uncharacteristically, he asked to go to see the doctor immediately. Dr. Kyeremateng referred him to emergency for suspected appendicitis; he was triaged at the Children's Hospital. Ultrasound showed a mass, but radiological consultation could not determine what was going on. It could have been appendicitis, they said, but, if so, it was presenting in an odd way. Debra advised them that Noah had had mesenteric adenitis a couple of years earlier, but they did not seem to think that explained the current problem.

I got a call to meet Debra at the Children's Hospital after work because nothing had yet been resolved, so Noah was to be admitted. With the doctors having decided against immediate emergency surgery, at least Noah was finally allowed to eat and drink, which he had not been able to do all that day. When I arrived at the hospital, everyone was concerned. Appendicitis still couldn't be ruled out, but neither was it a typical presentation if that's what it was. Nothing else could be ruled out either. All minds were reluctantly turning to cancer.

The next morning, after a long, painful night, Noah was sent for an MRI (at our request, in place of a CT scan, as we were reluctant to have him exposed to all that radiation), followed by the miserable experience of a barium swallow. And still, the doctors remained puzzled, unable to pinpoint what the problem was.

Of course, even among Lynch patients, it is almost unheard of for a 15-year-old to get colorectal cancer. But, at that point, we had not yet had Noah genetically tested, so it seemed to the doctors not only possible but even likely that he might be in the company of the youngest Lynch patients in Canada to get a colon tumour. Suddenly, in the space of an hour, we were told he apparently had bowel cancer, and his room filled with half a dozen specialists all waiting their turn to speak with us. After a buzz of consultation, the paediatric surgeon said Noah would be scheduled for a colon resection within a week, apologizing that it would take that long.

To us, there seemed nothing long about this process at all: the surgery pressed in with frightening rapidity. As stunned as we felt, though, we had been in this kind of pressure cooker before, so we started going through our paces, doing as we had always done. We pulled in Rob and began to research. We asked countless questions of the doctors, got copies of all test results, and recruited our friend Wendy to come in to the hospital and take notes as we reviewed, collated, and discussed all our information and defined and prioritized tasks. We educated the doctors about Lynch tumours and MSI (unfamiliar to the oncological fellow, we discovered), and we debated possible courses of action.

Throughout all of this, Noah was very strong but also very worried; he broke down crying at one point, just because it was all too much for him to bear. What 15-year-old could be expected to endure that? With the doctors trying to control his pain, he spent a couple of days in the hospital, always with Debra or me by his side. Debra would stay overnight with him, sleeping on the easy chair that pulled into a bed. He got sent home on the weekend for several days while we waited for his surgery date, and we met with the leadership in our church to have them pray for him, as the Bible tells believers to do.

It was time for us to grab hold of the lifeline that had been thrown out to us in February, 2008: we made a phone call to Spring Holter in Toronto, who connected us to Dr. Robert Gryfe, pre-eminent Lynch surgeon and researcher and a colleague of Drs. Gallinger and Moore. We were able to arrange a conference call between Dr. Gryfe in Toronto, Rob James in B.C., and ourselves and Noah's surgeon, Dr. Suyin Lum Min, in her office. There was thorough discussion about the various options. Once again, this second opinion had a direct impact on the course of Noah's treatment.

Rather than the immediate surgical resection of Noah's colon that had initially been planned, only investigative surgery would be pursued for the time being, it was concluded. If in fact the mass was confirmed not to be appendicitis, a biopsy would be performed, but nothing more radical. If pathology then revealed a malignancy, subsequent action would be reviewed at that point. The relief in putting off the radical surgery in favour of further investigation, so that as much information as possible could be collected and carefully examined in conjunction with the Toronto Lynch specialists before further action was taken, provided us immense relief. We were deeply grateful for Dr. Lum Min's gracious and collaborative spirit in allowing us to bring in Dr. Gryfe.

Noah's surgery took place on a Thursday, one week and one day after he had arrived at the emergency department. First, a paediatric gastroenterologist performed a gastroscopy and a colonoscopy, coming out to report to us that all was okay there. Then Dr. Lum Min performed laparoscopic surgery, looking first at the appendix to make sure all was well there, and then visualizing the mass that was outside Noah's colon, where she took a biopsy. Some alarm was raised at this point because, while Noah was confirmed not to have colorectal cancer, the doctor thought the mass might be lymphoma, which would have been a case of "out of the frying pan and into the fire."

Bless Dr. Lum Min; she made sure we got the fastest pathology report in Winnipeg history, so we did not have to agonize long. By mid-day Friday, she phoned us from an operating theatre, in the middle of another surgery she was performing, to tell us that Noah did not have cancer. His malady was likely an infection in the mesentery next to the colon, although she wasn't sure what had caused it. We were ecstatic.

Noah was to be checked out the following day, but not before suffering from a major medical miscommunication, coming at the hands of a misinformed and fairly tactless oncology fellow.

Later that Friday, I received a final call from Dr. Lum Min. Before I narrate the event in full, let me provide an aside about this fine specialist. She is, without a doubt, the nicest doctor I have ever met and a perfect person to be involved in paediatric medicine. As the surgeon in charge of Noah's treatment, she was responsible for being the project manager. So, she gathered paediatric oncologists and gastroenterologists around us. She became the point person for all of our questions and musings and was the brunt of our misgivings and potential over-reactions. We went to her many times with requests for second opinions and the involvement of other doctors, especially those whom we had in our circle from the Lynch centre in Toronto. Often we would approach her delicately, fearing she might be impatient with our endless questions or take offence at our requests. Instead, she graciously went out of her way to encourage us to bring forward every request and to voice every concern without any fear of offending her. Her attitude was the epitome of humility: the patient comes first, then the family, and finally her own ego. We loved her for that.

Only once was she irritated, and that was not with us: let me tell you what happened. A short time after getting the "all clear" as far as cancer was concerned, I received a final call from Dr. Lum Min once she had come out of surgery.

"Mr. Maione, I spoke briefly with Mrs. Maione this morning, as you'll know. I want to confirm that the pathologist has reported everything is clear. It is an infection, and Noah can go home soon. When the final pathology is done in a week, I can give him antibiotics."

"Yes, thank you so much, Dr. Lum Min. That is a huge relief."

After half an hour, I went to the nursing station to find out when I could take Noah home. Standing there was the oncology fellow we'd met in Noah's room during the surge of specialists who had crowded in after all the initial testing had led the doctors to a provisional diagnosis of cancer.

"Mr. Maione, glad I caught you. It seems that Noah has cancer, so we are going to start a chart at CancerCare, and the paediatric oncologist will be in touch with you as to treatment."

I paused. "I think you have your facts confused. I just had a conversation with Dr. Lum Min, who told me that he was clear. You might want to double check your information."

"I am not sure what she told you, but we are going to start a chart for him."

Irritated at this point, I retorted, "Start any chart you want; I am going to take him home now."

I walked back to Noah's room, where he was, once again, looking very worried and on the verge of tears.

"Did you hear all that?"

"Yeah, so ... do I have cancer?"

"No, the real doctor," I replied, emphasizing the word *real*, "said you are fine. But, I will give her a call just to be sure."

Walking out of the room, I called Dr. Lum Min.

"Dr. Lum Min, this is Dennis Maione. I just had a disturbing conversation with the oncology fellow, who tells me that Noah has cancer. I assured him that was not the case and suggested that perhaps he should get his facts straight before he takes any more action."

"This makes me very angry." (Her statement was ironic: not in its content, but by virtue of the manner in which she spoke. Dr. Lum Min is the gentlest, mildest-mannered person I have ever met. Her version of very angry is my reaction to cute kittens and puppies.)

"Can you give oncology a call to straighten things out? I will assume that you are correct unless I hear otherwise."

"Well, we no longer cane the residents, but I will ensure that this does not happen again."

The longer I thought about it, the more I thought that a few hours in stocks in the public square was just the remedy for his misdeed.

That evening, two Winnipeg Blue Bombers kindly stopped by Noah's bed on a visit through the ward. They chatted with him a bit and signed a hat and poster for him. Noah seemed pleased. After they'd left, he turned to me, "Wouldn't that have been neat if they'd been Saskatchewan Roughriders?" It had been five years earlier, while I'd lain in my hospital bed recovering from surgery, that Noah had been introduced to a love of football and, more specifically, the Saskatchewan Roughriders. A lot had happened since then, but this had not changed.

Before Noah left the hospital, a sample of his blood was obtained and sent for genetic testing for my Lynch mutation. It came back negative.

-28-

Postscript

A laugh's the wisest, easiest answer to all that's queer; ... I know not all that might be coming, but be it what it will, I'll go to it laughing.

Herman Melville, *Moby Dick*

That's the story so far. This ending seems a bit anticlimactic because, while there has been some relief, there has been no final life or death struggle, no heroic overcoming to bring closure. And, to be honest, I feel a bit of a fraud sometimes when I stand in the presence of people from whom cancer has taken so much more than it has taken from me.

For me, and for others who live with genetic predispositions to anything, especially diseases such as cancer, there is no end, really. There is day-to-day living, and every once in a while something comes up to challenge us; whenever that happens, we grit our teeth, and we do life even harder.

Since my second surgery things have changed. I decided, upon getting out of the hospital, that I was too fat and out of shape. So I started running. My first goal, in January of 2008, was to do a 10 km run in the summer. But that quickly became too small a goal, so I switched to a half marathon. In May of 2008, I ran my first half marathon, Debra cheering me on at the end with a large-lettered sign: "Guys without colons run faster!" I ran a second half marathon that fall, a third in the winter of 2009, and a fourth in the spring of 2009.

A year later, in the winter of 2010, I switched from distance running to triathlon events. At that time, still struggling with weight and fitness, I was 265 pounds. That summer I completed innumerable triathlons at sprint and Olympic distances. In winter of 2011, four years after my second surgery, I began training for my first half-Ironman distance, and I completed three half-Ironman distance races over the course of the summer. Not feeling that was a sufficient challenge, I hired a coach in the fall of 2011 and began training for my first full Ironman race. For those not familiar with the Ironman triathlon, the event includes a 3.8 km swim, followed by a 180 km cycle, and a 42.2 km run (a full marathon). I checked that off the list in the summer of 2012 in Penticton, British Columbia. The next year, in 2013, I completed my second Ironman race in Louisville Kentucky, bettering my previous time by a full hour. My race weight now hovers around 185 pounds.

Now, at (almost) 50, I am a full-time author and public speaker, having left a career in information technology, and I love my life. My son, Alex, and I just had our yearly scope (the first one for him), and we are both polyp- and cancer-free.

The spectre of cancer remains, and it will until the day that I die. Each year I will be forcefully reminded of its threat as I get my much beloved gastroscopy–sigmoidoscopy combination, and each year I wait for the "all clear" from Dr. Yaffe. Of course, there may be a time when what I hear is, "Dennis, I removed a polyp, and it's gone to pathology to be tested," or even, "Dennis, you have cancer," and I will start the dance all over again. But, who needs to worry about the might-bes? Today has enough problems, and more joys, of its own.

Part 2

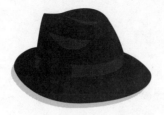

What I Learned
from Cancer

*I have undertaken, you see, to write
not only my life, but my opinions
also; hoping and expecting that your
knowledge of my character, and of
what kind of a mortal I am, by the
one, would give you a better relish
for the other: As you proceed further
with me, the slight acquaintance
which is now beginning betwixt
us, will grow into familiarity; and
that, unless one of us is in fault, will
terminate in friendship.*

Laurence Sterne,
The Life and Opinions of Tristam Shandy, Gentleman

-29-

A Part of the Main

No man is an island, entire of itself; every man is a piece of the continent, a part of the main. ... Any man's death diminishes me, because I am involved in mankind, and therefore never send to know for whom the bells tolls; it tolls for thee.

John Donne, "XVII. Meditation" in
Devotions upon Emergent Occasions

There is an episode of *Star Trek: The Next Generation* that I love, called "Tapestry." In it, the captain, Jean Luc Picard, is given a unique opportunity to change his past without affecting anyone or anything except himself. This opportunity is given him by an omnipotent being, Q, after Picard dies from a complication in his artificial heart, something that was implanted when he was a young man as the result of his arrogant misjudgement in a bar fight. In the episode, Picard applies his middle-aged wisdom to the situations in his early life and, based on that hard-won wisdom, changes a number of his decisions and actions, including the one that had caused the loss of his natural heart. However, after being returned to the present, now with his natural heart intact, along with other attendant consequences of his new actions, he finds that he is no longer the same, middle-aged person that he was. Rather than having become a wiser man as a result of learning from his younger self's quick, impulsive actions, he has become merely the product of someone who has always played it safe—in his words, a "dreary man in a dreary job." Thus, he petitions Q to put things back as they were before, and he eventually manages to recover from the situation that had initially caused his death. Picard then ponders all these events with his first officer. To paraphrase, he says, "There are a lot of things in my life that I regret: many events and circumstances that hung like loose threads from a tapestry. However, when I pulled some of those threads out, the whole thing simply unravelled."

For me, life is a tapestry, an existence full of threads. Some loose and some firmly woven in. In the course of writing my narrative, I discovered two of those firmly woven threads—threads which, if removed, would have changed the entire story.

These threads, the themes that I see, are two-fold: community and silence. First is the idea of the importance of community, both intentional and unintentional, organic and contrived, known and unknown. The community that formed around me during my illness and recovery was invaluable to me.

Second is the action of people in the silences of my narrative. I look back at the places in my story where there were gaps, places where I was asleep, either actually or metaphorically, and I see the movement in the darkness. As with the elves making shoes while the shoemaker slept, many things happened when I was not looking.

I will talk at length in a later chapter about community, but I want to introduce the idea here. So often we either overlook or dismiss outright the central importance of community. One of the reasons is the increasing individualization of our society and the isolation that comes from more of our needs being met without the need for personal interaction. The Internet has been a great source of convenience and, with a credit card and an Internet connection, there is very little, in terms of personal necessity, that I cannot get without having to leave my home. But at what cost? We have replaced the things that were real community with loosely connected pseudo-community such as Facebook can be. While those kinds of groups are, in many cases, valuable, they are second best to actually being in the same room as those whom you love and who love you. There is, after all, a reason that we feel disconnected from family and friends when they are away, even when they can call, email, and Skype: these are simply not replacements for the real thing.

I had a revelation during my my first cancer, a revelation of community. A revelation that came to me through first-hand experience, and one that I continue seeing played out crisis after crisis around me. I see community forming again and again out of nothing more than broken and often selfish individuals. During my first cancer, I was attending a church that was going through some significant problems, a crisis of vision and leadership. In that time, however, it came together for me, to support and love me, even though their problems with each other continued. I have often said of that time that the church became the church, if only briefly.

And we see that phenomenon occur time and time again:

communities come together around natural disasters, loss of life, or the diagnosis of critical or terminal illness. Somehow, during crisis people choose to set their differences and private concerns aside and come together to become all the community they can be. And then, almost inexplicably, but too often, community dissolves gradually thereafter, unable to hold itself together once the crisis has passed.

Cancer is crisis, and community is necessary. What follow are musings about being in and of community during cancer.

-30-

About Doctors

I will prescribe regimens for the good of my patients according to my ability and judgement and never do harm to anyone.

Excerpt from the *Hippocratic Oath*

In most societies and throughout history, doctors have been held in high regard, perceived with a certain amount of reverence, awe, and wonder. From the healer–priest and shaman voodoo practitioner to the family physician and surgeon, doctors are seen in a special light. After all, they know things the rest of us do not, and they have special, almost-seeming magical powers to restore health and to bring us back from the brink of death to life.

As Western society has evolved, medicine has become compartmentalized, and the role of the physician in the community has changed. While the doctor's role as counsellor and healer is still present in some corners, much of medicine has become business, so that the role of the doctor has shifted from generalized healer for all areas of life towards that of dispenser of medicines and fixer of medical problems. Of course, there are exceptions to this generalization, but it still is generally true.

This pressure to be the fixer of health problems has been magnified through a feedback loop that has developed. We are frustrated with medicine as business, we question whether life events such as birth and death should be treated as primarily medical situations, and we wonder how to get help with health and wellness, not just sickness. Consequently, we seek out alternative, so-called holistic practitioners to fill the gaps. Recognizing this as a threat to current medical practice, and in some cases being legitimately concerned about the efficacy and even safety of some alternative practices, many doctors put up walls and hold themselves up as the true scientific health care providers, the all-important evidence-based practitioners, and in so doing alienate the rest of the health care community.

The picture is changing, but ever so slowly. Midwives are now welcomed in some hospitals, acupuncture is offered by many physiotherapists, and limited chiropractic services are covered by public health care. Nonetheless, history bears out that the institution that is medicine stridently resists change.

While there has been some attempt to include alternative health care information in current medical education and practice, it is too often dealt with in a cursory way and even treated with disdain, almost like witchcraft. Furthermore, patients who want to look at additional therapies or bring new information to bear on an established practice or treatment—regardless of the source of that information in science or anecdote—are often treated with the same scepticism given to alternative practitioners.

The problem is that health practitioners—of all stripes—do not want to admit they have only part of the truth, that someone else might have legitimate independent insights or understanding.

So, who are doctors, these people who diagnose and cure our diseases? Well, simply put, regardless of their experience and expertise, doctors are people just like the rest of us. As a result, they are subject to all the same pressures as the rest of us, and to some extent, pressures that are magnified by the high expectations society has of them: to fix people, no matter what their ailments; to be patient and understanding, regardless of the patient's demeanour; and to be cool under pressure, regardless of what is at stake.

I know a lot of doctors: some of them are my specialists; some are my friends. I have a family doctor, a surgeon, an oncologist, and a cardiologist, all of whom I call "my" doctors. But I also have friends who are physicians: vascular surgeons, emergency doctors, and family practitioners.

Let me introduce you to my friend, Matt (not his real name). I have known Matt for more than 20 years. I met him when he was 14, a brash young man who had just broken up with his girlfriend and lamented that he would never find love, nor, of course, ever get married. Later, coming out of high school, Matt did four years pre-med, four years medical school, six years general surgery residency, and two years vascular surgery fellowship training. Now, I get to see Matt about once a year when he is in town for a conference. The last time I saw him, I asked, "Matt, how is doctoring going for you?"

Here is how he responded: "Well, Dennis, when I first started out in my own practice, I was terrified. Now, after 10 years, I'm finally at a place where I do not feel I'm going to make a dire mistake each time I step into the operating theatre."

Matt is a real person. He is a brilliant and skilled surgeon with years of training and years of experience. But, every time he steps into the operating theatre, he feels the weight of expectations. As the machines hiss and beep, and with his support staff around him, he often holds the lives of his patients in his hands. Matt has a wife and children, and he has the pressure of teaching daughters how to live in the world, sometimes with limited success. Matt is not arrogant—he cares for his patients—and he is not Superman; he is just a regular guy.

Data collected by the United States Centers for Disease Control in their 2013 National Occupational Mortality Surveillance (NOMS) program shows that, amongst Caucasian men and women (the group that currently represents the vast majority of doctors in North America), physicians have the highest rate of suicide and attempted suicide of all professions. Male doctors are almost twice as likely to attempt or commit suicide as men in other professions, and women almost three times as likely. This is presumably a consequence of the stress from expectations placed on them, both from the outside as well as from within themselves.

Why do I tell these stories and quote these statistics? Because it is important that we understand the strengths and failings of the people who care for us and that we act accordingly. It is as inappropriate to disregard their advice and treatment plans as it is to treat them as demi-gods who can do no wrong. So, here are some points of wisdom that I can share regarding doctors.

Recognize that your doctor will have good and bad days.

Just as one angry outburst at your spouse does not make you a bad husband or wife, one bad experience with your doctor does not make her a bad doctor; it just makes her a real person.

Recognize that your doctor, the one who has the formal medical training, possesses a certain skill set but may be insecure (perhaps not overtly) about stretching those boundaries—for example, about your bringing forward knowledge or about including alternative providers in your healing.

Like it or not, many people no longer have blind faith in their doctors; we want them to earn our trust, especially at the critical junctures of our health care. I think it is perfectly appropriate to use all the expertise at your disposal to help your body get well. Despite having a scientific bent to my outlook on life, I see no inherent problem in mixing surgery with prayer and exercise and natural remedies, as long as everyone you are consulting knows all the things you are doing. Unfortunately, problems can arise when natural medicines (or even more common substances from the shelves of stores) have bad reactions with pharmaceutical drugs. Did you know, for example, that grapefruit can interact negatively with at least 85 prescription drugs—with at least 44 of those being potentially fatal? Grapefruit increases the effectiveness of drugs, thus leading to unintentional overdose and toxicity: some pharmaceutical drug effects are magnified 20 times when taken with as little as 200 ml of grapefruit juice. So, if you are going to go on a juice fast while taking chemotherapy, let your oncologist know, so she can help you anticipate the possible side effects of your actions.

Some doctors will embrace alternative–holistic healing methods, either welcoming the efficacy of these treatments, or, at the very least, tolerating those which are innocuous or are psychologically beneficial even when not physically beneficial. Other physicians will be hesitant and will need to be won over. Many will submit to your desire and the demands you make for additional help, but all doctors will need to feel as though you are including them in your process.

Recognize that your doctor has feelings that can be hurt and an ego that can be bruised.

I was in Dr. Yaffe's examining room one day, getting a routine examination after he'd fixed a hernia that probably resulted from overexertion after my second cancer surgery. I happened to mention to him that my brother-in-law and I had been talking about both of us being scheduled for the same upcoming procedure, but that his doctor was going to use laparoscopy and had cited the method Dr. Yaffe was going to use for me as "old school." I tossed off this comment fairly casually, not considering at all that it might be offensive. Dr. Yaffe retorted, with some irritation in his voice, "I could have done that procedure; however, given the amount of scarring your abdomen has already experienced, I did not want to take any chances with my ability to fix you properly: it was not 'old school'; it was a clinical choice." I had never heard him irritated before, but I could tell that he had taken offence at having his decision questioned, especially by someone who was evaluating his technique out of context. Our relationships with our care givers are just that: relationships. And, as such, we all have an obligation to conduct ourselves with civility and consideration.

Remember that you have the right to the best medical care and that you deserve to be heard and respected.

For all the talking that I have done about respecting the personhood of doctors, I have to make it clear that they are not always right and that, whether for the sake of expedience or something else, they can forcefully assert their therapeutic direction seemingly without acknowledgement of the patient's wishes or feelings. Of course, this stark contrast to their expert caregiving role is also due to their being real people, but that fallibility is not an excuse. As long as you remain reasonable in your demands of them, you have the right to expect they be reasonable and gracious in their response to you. I use the word *reasonable* very specifically because I know patients (who are just as real and therefore fallible) who can be very unreasonable. When that happens, I see no reason why a doctor cannot release that patient "to find another health care provider who is better able to meet their needs."

So, if you are confused about your diagnosis or your treatment plan, you have the right to ask questions and be heard: to fully understand what is wrong with you, what will be done to fix you, and what the short- and long-term implications are. If you are paying for your treatment, you also have a right to know how much it's going to cost, how payments must be made, and whether your insurance is going to cover it (thankfully, as a Canadian, I do not have to worry about this, for the most part). And, finally, if you are not comfortable with your doctor, you have the right to ask for a second opinion and/or for a referral to another doctor.

31

About Community

What do we live for, if it is not to make life less difficult for each other?

George Eliot, *Middlemarch*

As a teenager in the '80s, I could not help but be influenced by the movies of John Hughes, including the iconic *The Breakfast Club*. In it, five teens, all from different demographics, are compelled to spend a Saturday together in the school library, the result of various detention-warranting offences. Through their shared experience, they find a level of commonality and community that none of them could have expected. Initially blinded by the filters of their own lives and experience, the stereotypical responses they begin with soon crumble as they see the humanity within each other. And by the end of that day, they are a group, if bonded only for a short time by shared experience and new insight into each other. Brought together, they find out the whole is greater than the several parts they represent: brain, athlete, basket case, princess, and criminal.

Throughout this book, I have stressed the need for community. This I do unapologetically because it is the most profoundly significant asset that you have. This community will provide you with care, support, prayer, advice, and companionship throughout your journey through cancer. No one should go through cancer alone, and no one should have to manage all of the intricacies of the process using solely their own emotional fortitude, brains, or practical resources. I know that some people have difficulty with this, and their first response to trauma is to withdraw. I understand that. Know, however, that there are people who love you and want to help, and all it may take is a small push to get that ball rolling. You do not need to become an extrovert in order to build community and rely on it. In fact, if it makes you more comfortable, ask someone else to build it for you, and have them ensure that most of what is done is behind the scenes.

A cancer diagnosis can be profoundly distressing and psychological damaging. However, I encourage you, before fear, uncertainty, and treatment take their toll on you, to gather your community around you, or designate someone to gather it for you. While your community may form organically and unbidden, do not take for granted that it will. Often, people will not volunteer for the jobs you need them to do without your asking—not because they do not want to help, but because they might feel uncomfortable asking what you need and even less comfortable presuming to tell you what they can provide. But you need these people: the project manager, bodyguard, comedian, social convenor, spiritual director, athlete, medical coordinator, researcher, and biographer. While some people may fill more than one of these roles, it is very difficult for one person to be all of these things and even more difficult to be all of them on a full-time basis. Try not to see your spouse or significant other as the end-all and be-all of your support, no matter what kind of a person he or she is. Not only will your care be compromised, but it is likely that he or she will burn out in the process.

So, make a community. Gather the people you need and let them know what their roles are. Let the comedian know that her job is to do funny things, bring funny movies, and take you to comedy clubs. Let her know that she has no other responsibilities and that she need not feel guilty about her limited role: it is an important one. The same holds true for the athlete, who helps you maintain some activity in your life, and the social convener, the spiritual director, the chef, the bookworm, the scientist, and all the other people whom you are going to draw around you to provide you with support.

I really like lists, as they help me to remember things. My wife and kids maintain that I have a mind like a sieve, and they really are right. I can remember the one thing currently on my mind, but if I do not make lists and write other things down, those things are soon gone.

So, I will make you a list. This list is not exhaustive; on the other hand, not every item may be applicable to you. The point of this list is to acknowledge there are certain things cancer patients need to do or to have done for them. It is useful first to identify your needs and then to create a job title and description so as to get each of those needs met. In this way, things get done, and it's easier to distribute the burden over a number of people rather than looking to one individual to take care of everything.

Here are some of the roles you should consider making a part of your community:

1) Project Manager
2) Bodyguard
3) Comedian
4) Social Convener
5) Chef
6) Spiritual Director
7) Athlete
8) Medical Coordinator
9) Researcher
10) Biographer

Of course, I am not implying that because you have cancer, you are somehow debilitated and completely unable to care for yourself. That is not the truth at all. However, things that happen during stressful situations can move people from complete self-sufficiency to a state of greater dependency. This can range from one's complete inability to cope to the simple neglect of certain areas that easily get overlooked or de-prioritized in the wave of trauma that overwhelms you. In addition, there are certain physical factors that come into play because of therapy. Medication can make some things difficult: chemotherapy patients often complain of "brain fog"—that feeling that you are just not quite all there. Pain medication may also serve to incapacitate you, both mentally and physically. Finally, the exhaustion of treatment and recovery means that you may not always have the wherewithal to manage everything in your life.

You are a whole person, with the needs of a whole person. The reality is that when you get sick, many of your needs take a back seat to the feeling that you just need to get yourself well. However, cancer is not like the 24-hour flu, either in its severity or impact. And recovery from cancer is not something you can just leave your whole life behind to deal with; you continue to have needs, and those needs must be met.

I have identified these roles because they represent areas of your life that need to be taken care of—fostered really—while you and your doctors are dealing with your cancer. And they are areas of your life that have the possibility of slipping through the cracks. You should not treat these things as optional: you cannot simply replace good food with pizza pops, for example, and assume that your recovery will be just as good as if you had not (my apologies to anyone for whom pizza pops has been the only thing you could keep down during chemo).

I focus here on community because when you do not have the

strength to do these things, your community can take over for you to ensure that your whole person is being taken care of. When you do not have the ability to find laughter on your own, your comedian can be there to pick up the slack. When you feel restless but do not know what to do, your athlete can go for a walk with you or accompany you outside to play with your dog. In fact, in the guise of cancer treatment, you may find you can foster the kind of whole-life, healthy lifestyle that you never had before.

Remember that not all roles will be equally important at all times. But it is best to have people available to you to take over when you are not able. Also, be sure that you spread these roles out over your support group. No one person has the capacity to manage all these roles for you, and it is unfair to expect that one person can. Finally, think about continuing this through your post-cancer life; new things and new ideas can often be good for the soul.

Be intentional about this. I encourage you to identify people who can fill these roles and then to actually sit down with them and say something like this: "Joe, the next six months are going to be hard for me, and I am not always going to be able to have fun or take the time to find funny things, but I need that. I am hoping you can take on the role of comedian for me. If you accept this role, I will look to you to keep fun in my life. While I do not expect you to be available 24 hours a day, what I'm hoping is that you can commit an hour a week to help me out. Find me funny books to read or TV shows or movies to watch."

If you can be clear about what you need and expect, then people will be more willing to commit to helping you out. This may seem very managed or forced, but it does not have to be. If you need something, it's better to have it planned out and be certain it will happen than to wait for spontaneous things, only to have nothing at all happen.

The Project Manager

You need someone to take care of everything. Not to do it all, but to be sure that everything is coordinated. Of course, you can do this yourself, but if you are recovering from cancer, or you are in treatment, you might find this overwhelming. It's nice to have someone with a pencil and clipboard to keep track of the whens and wheres of everything you do, the priority of the whats you have to do, and the contact information for people involved. It's amazing how many things need to get done when you have "nothing" to do. There are medical appointments, people you need to see, and people who need to see you. Having someone to remind you of all of these things and to trouble-shoot logistical problems is indispensable. This role is best filled by someone who has close access to your schedule and insight into you and your life. A significant other or a close friend can be the best one to help out because some of the things are going to be personal enough that you don't want to share them with the world.

The Bodyguard

He stands in the corner with a hat, dark glasses, a trench coat, and a radio in his ear. He has a slight bulge on the left under his coat that could be a gun or a tuna-fish sandwich. He is your bodyguard.

Okay, maybe that's the wrong image, but I need to make something clear. Your bodyguard knows your schedule, when you are tired, and when you are lively. She knows you need to keep your strength up for the time when your sister is going to visit, and she tells people they cannot see you this day. Your bodyguard is the one who controls others' access to you, especially during periods when you can easily be found by all the well-meaning people who want to visit you. Her protection is particularly needed when you are in the hospital or confined to your bed at home.

While unfettered access to you might seem like a good idea when you are feeling perky, there will be a lot of times during your recovery when that is not the case. Surgery is tiring, drugs are tiring, chemotherapy is tiring, and people are tiring, especially if you are an introvert. Even extroverts will find that their very nature causes interactions which sap their strength and leave them wondering how they ever managed so many relationships in the past. So have someone who can stop people at the door to your hospital room or at the door to your home and say, "Susan is not up to seeing anyone right now. Here is my mobile number; text me later, and I'll let you know if she is feeling stronger then." (Of course, if your name is not Susan, you might want to have your bodyguard use your name; otherwise, people will be very confused.)

The point here is that someone else, not you, needs to manage your social calendar when you are weak or feeling ill. Not all have the sensitivity to recognize when you are exhausted but putting on a game face to make them feel welcome. Not everyone can hear the subtext, "Please go now; I am worn out" when you say, "Well, my kids are going to be here soon," or "I should get ready for supper now." Someone to make those requests explicit is invaluable.

When I was hospitalized the first time, I had no bodyguard. Debra was working in a different city, and most of my friends and family had daytime jobs. So, not only was I alone throughout the day, but I was also unprotected. Let me be clear, I could not be more grateful for the people who came to visit me when I was hospitalized. Like many things, however, too much, even of a really good thing, can be overwhelming.

I recall one friend who came to visit in the mid-afternoon. I had not seen him for a while, and he was going through some difficult times. So, for about an hour, we talked. By the time he left, I was exhausted. The kind of exhausted that means within five minutes of his leaving, I was fast asleep. Another of my friends showed up about 30 minutes later, however, and I awoke with a start, dazed and confused about where I was, what I was doing there, and who this guy in my room was. It was a difficult visit.

The bodyguard can help you by ensuring that access is controlled, so that encouraging interactions are just that, rather than events to be recovered from. He could even make a sign for you to put up in your room, "I'm tired today; please keep your visits to 10 minutes or less." That way, expectations get set at the outset of the visit. Of course, you can also be your own bodyguard by protecting your time and letting people know gently but firmly when it is time for them to leave because you need to rest.

The Comedian

Laughter is not only an indication that you are having fun; it also has both short- and long-term physiological benefits. It may seem obvious that if you are laughing, the emotion of happiness is foremost in your mind. There is more, though. The chemicals released in your body during laughter have further effects: pain-killing properties, blood-pressure lowering properties, and the long-term benefit of helping boost the body's ability to heal itself. They help keep depression away.

So, get funny! Or expose yourself to laughter, to funny things and people. These days, funny is easy to find. You do not need to go out to find it, although you can. You can play funny on your Blue Ray, you can stream funny on your computer or phone, and you can even do funny with your friends. Cancer is not a funny thing, but funny can be your release, if only for a moment, from the seriousness of cancer.

Expose yourself to really funny things every day. I'd recommend 30 minutes, if you can manage it. Find a situation comedy or comedian you really like and laugh. What you find funny is a personal thing, so I'm not going to try to create a definitive list. I love British comedy, and that would be high on my list. Make a list of your own favourites, and see what kinds of creative ways you, your friends, or family can come up with to help you get access to the things on your list.

Find time to spend with enjoyable and funny people. Do you have a friend who is a laugh a minute? Can he suspend his concern over your cancer enough to laugh with you the way you laughed before you got sick? Can he help you joke through the serious subjects? He may not be the deep-thought guy, but you do not need that from him. Plan to spend time with him every week. If he is creative, maybe he'll compile a video or a Facebook slideshow of cat pictures to show you.

Do funny in the company of others. Ever notice how things are funnier when you're together with others than when you're alone? Getting out to enjoy humour can enhance the experience as well as serve to get you away from your normal routine. When I was in hospital the first time, I was given a pass to get out and be social with my friends. As long as there is not a problem with your being away from medical care, I would suggest you do this. You will feel better for the experience.

The Social Convener

Get out when you can. Sometimes this is connected with your comedian, but other times it just means escaping from the mundane world you have found yourself in and getting a change of scenery. This is not always easy. Sometimes you are going to feel really sick, especially if you are in the middle of chemo, but leave it to your social convener and project manager to help you out. The latter should know your treatment schedule, when you typically feel the best, and when you might be feeling up to an outing or getting together with friends.

The Chef

Remember to eat, and eat well. Once again, chemotherapy raises its ugly head and conspires against you to make you despise all food. But you do have to eat, so try to eat well. Get your chef to make you nutritious meals you can hold down. He might work with a dietician to create meals that are palatable to you and contain what your body needs.

The Spiritual Director

I know that not everyone who reads this has the same idea of spirituality. I hope that amongst my readers are Christians, Muslims, Buddhists, Pagans, Atheists, Agnostics, and all other manner of *-ians* and *-ists*. In the spirit of full disclosure, I will tell you that I am a Christian, and it is from within that faith, relationship, and worldview that I speak and write. However, ensuring that the spiritual component of your life is cared for while you are dealing with cancer is not specifically Christian; in fact, it is not a uniquely religious thing at all. It is a quest to ensure that the intangible part of you which cannot be seen, felt, or quantified is cared for. For me, it is easier to speak in the context of my relationship with God as I try to explain the importance of this role: personal prayer, community prayer, and the quest for the direct intervention of God in my life and my healing. Receive and adjust this advice as your worldview mandates or allows, but do not let that part of you wither away during cancer treatment and recovery; it may be the only part that is capable of staying resilient during such a time.

If you are a friend or family member of a cancer patient, be both bold and sensitive in your approach to spirituality. Generously offer what you can in terms of spiritual support, but do not push or use this crisis as an excuse to proselytize. If your friend rejects your offers, find other ways to feed that spiritual need.

The Athlete

Don't neglect your body in the midst of your crisis. You may not (or *may*) be able to run a marathon, but I would encourage you to walk around the block when you can. In August, 2013, I ran an Ironman race in Louisville, Kentucky. That weekend, a Canadian woman participated in the same race in Whistler, B.C. What made her feat remarkable is that she was undergoing chemotherapy for pancreatic cancer at the time. While I would not recommend such a fitness regimen while in active treatment, it goes to show that it is possible to maintain an outstanding level of fitness while on chemo.

Find a partner to do fitness things with. It might be your spouse, or it might be a friend, but do get up and out when you are able.

The Medical Coordinator

Someone needs to keep track of the people who care for you. Both in the hospital and out, there will be an array of doctors and care givers who will treat you, all with their own specialties and expertise. It will probably be the case that one doctor will take the lead in your care, but it remains important to sort out who is who, and what each is responsible for. In addition, there may be medical residents who fill in for the primary care providers, at least on an occasional basis. They need to be identified as well, and your medical coordinator—or you, if you don't have one—needs to find out their level of autonomy: are they making their own decisions or deferring to someone more senior in their specialty?

In addition, in the hospital there will be a number of nurses charged with your care. Again, your medical coordinator should get to know who they are, treat them well, and help you with this. Nurses are the most under-appreciated group of medical care givers in our society, and their contribution demands our appreciation and respect.

When you leave the hospital, things can get a bit more chaotic, especially if you are getting follow-up treatment from a number of different sources. Someone needs to track who is doing what and when those things are happening. If you are getting chemotherapy or are on medication for your pain, do not leave the minutia of your schedule to your own brain because, as I have found, that will invariably fail you sooner or later. Find someone who can keep track of these things for you, so you do not have to expend energy on them.

The Researcher

Doctors do not always have the time or resources to stay abreast of all the current research. This is especially the case if your cancer has presented strangely or is unusual in any way. As a result, you should do two things: first, talk to your doctors about working together with you as you dig up research; and two, find someone to help you out with this. The first point may help you prevent or overcome any potential resistance your care givers may show in response to your coming to them with new information or even extensive questions about your treatment. Let them know what journals or other web sites you are consulting, and ask for their input and guidance. In this way, it will feel less of an ambush when you arrive with a handful of journal articles from which you have discerned your own optimal treatment plan outside of the experience and knowledge of your doctors. A sudden deluge of information, no matter how scientific, combined with your own strong ideas of how that could be applied in your case, will generally not be received well.

Getting someone to help you out, especially someone with scientific expertise and medical knowledge, will be invaluable as you try to sift the good information from the excellent information. When I was contemplating the options for follow-up from my second cancer, my friend Rob did a lot of research with my wife, Debra, on Lynch syndrome and the treatment options that were available. Much of the research was new. And all of it was full of statistical information, laden with terms such as *sample sizes, multivariate analysis, double-blind studies,* and *survival rates.* In many cases, I could not make heads or tails of what the authors were trying to say about the efficacy of one treatment over another. Rob, however, has expertise in the interpretation of statistical information, and this was invaluable as we wended our way through the data. See if you can find a doctor who is not involved in your care (a friend or perhaps your family practitioner) to help you understand the jargon and technical talk that comes with medical literature. Again, this will be invaluable as you try to determine the information you want to bring forward to your care providers.

The Biographer

Here is what I discovered in looking back over my cancer and its treatment: there are significant things I wish I could now remember better—or even at all. I wish I could remember more clearly the people who visited me and what they said. I wish that my mind's eye possessed a clear vision of all of the events. I wish that I'd had a biographer, someone to record all these things for me.

When I was in hospital the second time, Debra and I set up two practices that helped us: (1) we had a scrapbook we used as a combination memory keeper and visitor's log; and (2) Debra posted updates on my care and condition on a web site called Carepages, a place where people could also leave messages of encouragement for me. My hospital guests were invited to record their visit in a scrapbook with blank pages, into which we also taped the many cards received from well wishers. We had a large set of coloured pens available to encourage people's creativity and to help them relax. (This also gave them something to do, reducing the pressure on me to entertain them.) In addition, we took a digital photo of everyone who came to visit me, which we later printed and included in the scrapbook. Rather than have everything in a digital format, we wanted a tangible memento of the generous caring we were recipients of.

Carepages gave us an online presence for people near and far who wanted to stay abreast of my situation but who could neither talk to us directly nor visit in person. This tool also provided a highly efficient way for Debra to keep family and friends informed without having to expend vast amounts of energy to contact everyone individually. These days, similar websites, Facebook, and other social media offer further tools to choose from.

A good friend of mine recently had pancreatic cancer and, after a short but intense struggle, died only a few months after his diagnosis. In order to keep people up to date while dealing with the growing pressure of providing support and palliative care to her husband, his wife used Facebook to post information. This virtual space developed into a place for their family to share events and photos and for his friends to pay tribute, remember better times, and console the family and each other. It became, for a short while, a living community of help and support. I regret that I did not make copies of some of its rich content before the page was closed down after his death.

Remembering is important, but who is going to do it? This may happen spontaneously via a Facebook page, or you may want to be more intentional or far-reaching in planning for this. For example, you could keep your own written journal of thoughts and feelings. These days, digital cameras and video are virtually everywhere, so be creative and make use of them. Some people keep video journals in order to make it easier. Others find it cathartic to be able to arrange their own memorial, to craft something that best expresses them. This could contain video, images, artifacts, and writing, which could come from you or from your friends and family. Some people like to be public with this sort of thing, and others prefer to be private. Together with your appointed biographer, you can control the tone and extent of the documentation of your experience and the memorializing of your life.

Let me conclude with this. My uncle and aunt are ranchers in southern Alberta. They live in a house they built with their own hands. Well, that is not quite true. They envisioned the project, but the house itself was built with quite a few hands. Running the length of the structure is a huge wooden beam, and if you look closely at it, you will see many burn marks—the brands of other ranchers in the area who helped them put that massive beam into place.

As a North American, I live in a very individualistic society, one that has been fashioned after the idea that we stand alone, we live and die alone, we claw and scrape for everything we have, and that in order for the fruits of those labours to mean anything, they must be achieved alone. I have to admit that I have bought into that lie too many times throughout my life.

In reality, however, my life is a house, erected over many years, in which every experience I've had is reflected. In the middle of that house is a beam, one that bears the marks of those people whose contributions have been branded into my life. These marks represent people without whom I could not have lived or loved, people who are a constant reminder that I am never really alone in my pain or joy.

32

About Advocacy

And I must continue to follow the path I take now. If I do nothing, if I study nothing, if I cease searching, then, woe is me, I am lost. That is how I look at it—keep going, keep going come what may.

Vincent Van Gogh, in a letter to his brother Theo (1880)

Sometimes I like to think about the ideal world. The utopia where we can trust that people and systems will always function in the most reasonable manner, where every great behemoth of an organization functions with the intelligence and thoughtfulness of the Canadian Parliament ... . Wait! Sorry, I think that last bit was just fantasy, too.

In my ideal world, when I get sick—if that even happens—my doctor has a lot of time to discuss my history and my risk factors. She does all the necessary tests quickly, consults all the medical literature, and is able to bring a highly skilled team around her to diagnose my illness and come up with the perfect strategy, unique to me and my situation, which will make me as well as I can get. In the ideal world, my doctor is my medical project manager, and I can leave everything in her capable hands and just show up at the meetings I'm scheduled to attend.

But, there is no ideal world. Doctors are overworked because there are too many sick people and not enough care givers to go around: as the population ages, this is only going to worsen. In addition, our personal health care is fragmented, split between our family doctors (if we are fortunate to have one), walk-in clinics, hospital emergency rooms, specialists, and a bevy of alternative and complementary practitioners. As a result, my doctor may not know everything that is going on with my body, nor the conditions affecting it, and, furthermore, may not have the time to work out all the implications of various treatments, even if she has been able to keep up with all the current clinical practices. So, I am left to manage my own health and health care, coordinating each of my doctors or specialists assigned to a specific body part or group of parts. In the end, the quality of my health care is a function not only of the quality of the health care system, but also of a measure of luck—having a doctor who happens to know just the right thing at just the right time. Its quality is also a function of the time and effort I am able to put into it.

Does this sound daunting? It certainly was for me. Until the first time I had rectal bleeding and was subsequently diagnosed with cancer, I had seen only one doctor in the decade since I was a teenager—with the exception of the several emergency room doctors who had given me stitches or treated my tree-planting injuries. So, when I casually entered a walk-in clinic to consult a doctor because I was having bleeding that I could not account for, I had no idea of the journey of frustration and discovery I was embarking on.

What I learned above all else was that I am my own best advocate. I am the one who makes the decisions; I, with my team, am the one who weighs the evidence; I am the one who chooses whether to simply take what my medical practitioners say and accept it at face value or to ask thoughtful questions until there are no nagging worries, doubts, or information gaps remaining. Often, I am the one to seek out a second informed opinion, as this is not something our health care system encourages as a matter of course. It is interesting to note, by the way, that doctors who themselves are ill tend to be the first to seek out second and even third and fourth opinions.

In both instances that I got cancer, I ended up making significant decisions outside the context of the original physician assigned to me. In the first instance, my decision-making process began with, "This does not sound right to me," and moved quickly to consulting a trusted mentor who was also a medical professional. In the second instance, I worked together with friends of considerable expertise to find expert guidance on whether to proceed with chemotherapy. In both cases, I had to doggedly pursue outside resources to get questions answered and, even then, some of what I decided was just my best guess. I have realized over the years that medicine is as much an art as a science and not nearly the pure science that some believe it to be.

So what does this mean for the average person? I've remarked more than once to my friends and family that I cannot imagine how things would have turned out had I not had resources at my finger tips to deal with my illness, its proposed treatments, my anxiety, and my confusion. I had a good education and a relatively stable home life, and I have tried to stay well read and well informed throughout my life. I have also maintained wide circles of friends who have afforded me expertise in a variety of crises, individuals all available through a phone call or an email. My outcomes would have been vastly different had I grown up disadvantaged, known no doctors, or lacked the self-confidence to challenge some of the opinions and advice I received.

If I were starting this process all over again, what would I tell myself? Here are some things I believe are important.

Become comfortable with your health care provider(s).

A good rapport with all your health care providers, especially your primary care giver, is of utmost importance. You need to be able to talk with this person, hear what he is saying, and evaluate what you hear. You cannot afford to have this process clouded by thoughts such as, "What a jerk he is," or, "I wonder if she has ever done this procedure before?" Think of your doctor as the person you are hiring to fix your roof or your car. Yes, the expertise is different, and, yes, the stakes are much higher, but, in the end, this person is going to get your consent to do life-altering things to your body, and you need to feel good about that person and what she is telling you.

Understand and be involved, but do not micromanage the process.

When I go to get my hair cut, I usually just walk in and say, "Make it look good." I like to approach professionals that way in general because, in the end, they are the ones with the expertise, and they know more about what they are doing than I do. Sometimes I go as far as to say, "I like this—can you do that?" or "Make me look like Brad Pitt." (Generally, I smile after that: no one is going to make me look like Brad Pitt!) I sometimes know what I want; I generally do not know how to get there.

Medical care can be like that. But while you ought not micromanage, you should know what is going to happen and why, so that you can give informed consent. Nevertheless, be sensitive to the fine line between being involved and micromanaging. Once you've decided on the course of action and the practitioner you approve of, it's time to stand aside and let the doctor do her work.

Find advocacy groups that can help you.

It seems I'm back to talking about community again. There is no point reinventing any wheels if someone has already done that work for you. All national cancer groups have local chapters in most major centres, and these are populated with staff and volunteers waiting for you to ask for their help. In addition, there may be groups to support people just like you, whether that is you with your specific cancer, financial circumstance, or family situation. There are also many online groups dedicated to bringing together people facing the same challenges.

At the heart of advocacy is support: support for you in your life, your circumstance, your cancer. Sometimes advocacy means that you stand up and saying, "This feels out of control, and I need some help to sort it out." Sometimes advocacy involves a call to a local cancer agency to ask someone to come and help you talk to your doctor. In the end, advocacy results in your getting the treatment you need from a system that can otherwise be impersonal and seem to forget about you.

-33-

About Dying

Because I could not stop for Death—
He kindly stopped for me—
The Carriage held but just ourselves—
And Immortality.

Emily Dickinson, "The Carriage" in *Poems: Series 1*

Wouldn't it be grand? A world where no one gets sick, no one grows old, no one gets cancer, and no one ever dies. I walk out into the bright sunlight on a summer's day, feel the breeze on my face, and hear the birds sing. I lie in the grass and hear the stream running by me, and I think to myself, "Life is good." And on those days it seems as though nothing can go wrong, and everything will be okay.

But it's not going to be okay. The world is not okay, and the same sun that shines down on me and causes me joy beats down on the African continent and causes drought and starvation. Some might even argue that the very leisure I enjoy has been obtained on the backs of the poor and the down-trodden.

It's not going to be okay. Steve Jobs got pancreatic cancer and had an arsenal at his disposal to fight it: a virtually unlimited budget for custom DNA sequencing for tumour-tailored chemotherapy, along with the best research, top doctors, and most powerful nutritional supplements to be had—all of which quite probably prolonged his days. In the end, however, he could not beat the disease that took his life.

It's not going to be okay. Not if your idea of okay is physical life without end or interruption. Because for all of us, life will be interrupted; we all die. Whether you believe that this life is strictly material or has a spiritual dimension, and regardless of your ideas about the possibility or nature of an afterlife, this physical existence is going to end.

"It's going to be okay." We so desperately want to hear those words at many times and in many circumstances throughout our lives. Through sickness, through health, through aging, we want to be reassured that this time is not the last time, that it's going to be okay. But it's not going to be okay if an infinite extension of life is what you are looking for.

Yet, it is going to be okay. I believe in hope; I believe that, in some real sense, everything is going to be okay. At the same time, I also know that mortality is a reality built into our DNA, (ironically, cancer cells function exactly as though the opposite is true, propagating without limit). So, we live in the tension between being alive, vibrant, and full of hope, and the reality, realized or not, that one day we are all going to die. Despite the hope you may derive from the prospect of living, or of not being, beyond the grave (depending on your religious beliefs), there remains a human ache that comes in any moment of stark realization that there will be a time when we are not here, when we will not have our friends and family and lovers to lean on or to watch and cheer as they grow and develop, fail and succeed.

As I age, I watch the generations of the family I have known and loved disappear. And although my parents are still alive, as are those of my wife, I am at the age where I am seeing the generation before them being taken one at a time. These are the grandparents, the great-aunts and -uncles, and even the siblings of my parents. Only recently I watched my wife's grandmother, our Oma, come to the end of her 101-year life. And while we were sad at her passing, not one of us commented that her life had been too short or her death untimely, with so much undone and left to accomplish. I recall Oma saying on more than one occasion that she wanted to "go home." Not to leave the nursing home and move back to the apartment she had shared with her husband of 72 years, but to leave the earth to be with Jesus. And while we were sad anticipating her loss, we all grieved over her pain and prayed for that fulfillment of her deepest longing.

But untimely death is not like that. When we encounter the death of any child, we weep over the loss because it affects us personally. We weep over the lost potential as we see taken from us a future artist or scientist, a world-changer. We experience the death of a young adult, and we mourn the loss of his development, compassion, vigour, and drive to succeed. We are moved by the death of the middle-aged as we look back over their lives and realize that either there was much more of the same to come, or that they were just ready to turn a corner to new beginnings. In all of these situations, we mourn the life cut short.

I am a triathlete. I am competitive in the sense that I have an interest in how well I do, in whether I am improving, and, with some assertion of ego, in whom I beat. While I will never win an event, I do not race simply to finish; I race to do well, as well as I can. However, it is telling that when I reflect on what I like about training and racing, it is really the finishing that I enjoy the most. The part when I can see the end goal, and, digging deep for a burst of energy I didn't think I possessed, I finish—and finish well. Then, with pride, I find myself able to say, "I did this task, and I did it well." Regardless of how I feel upon completion, however, I realize that the quality of the finish is a product of the quality of my training. Poor training means poor performance, and that means a bad feeling upon completion, the kind of regret that says, "If only I had applied myself in that situation, I would have had a better result."

Life, I have discovered, is like that. We all want to finish well, to get to the end with the sense that we have trained well. Also that, having lived well, we can have a "good death." It is important at this point for me to be clear that, in my opinion, having a good death has nothing to do with the absence of pain or stress. The most fulfilling life, I would submit, begins with an objectively good life and ends with a good death. However, a good death can end a bad life, and a bad death can end a good life. Sometimes we have the opportunity to evaluate our own life and impending end, and sometimes those labels of good and bad are applied by those whom we leave behind; at any rate, the most we can do is our best to ensure that both our life and death are good.

My friend Reg lived life well. But at 56, having endured the ravages of pancreatic cancer for eight months, he died. Reg loved life; he loved the challenges that it provided. He loved his wife, his daughters, his friends, his family, his students, and even his casual acquaintances. He loved to hear stories, perhaps as a way to experience life from the perspective of others, a way to expand the breadth of his own life. And he loved to tell stories. But cancer took all of this, all that he was. His body, sturdy and strong, was reduced to a virtual skeleton, literally a small fraction of what it had been. His mind, always as sharp as a whip and brilliant, was dulled by the brain fog of chemotherapy, eventually becoming only a reflection of his former wit and intellect.

We, the people he left behind when he died, wept and lamented the shortness of his life. The prematurity of his exit. The unfairness of it all. The lost potential. We measured the length of his days, and we found them to be insufficient. At first, we were overwhelmed because we felt he was cheated. As time has passed, we feel that most of all we have been cheated: of his presence, his wisdom, and even his horrible puns. But, despite our resentment of "life" or "fate" or "God," I cannot help but reflect on what Reg said about his life: "I have had a good run, and, while I would have liked more time, I had a pretty good life." This was not the resignation of a man who was angry or depressed at a fate he could not control, but rather the acknowledgement of one who knew that he had run his race to completion and it was now time for him to stop. He had lived a good life, and he was able to die a good death.

From my experience and that of others around me, I have learned some things about life and death.

I have learned, first and foremost, that life is meant to be lived.
This idea is summed up In the Latin phrase *vive ut vivas*, which means, "Live so that you may live." There is nothing more tragic than seeing a wasted life, whatever that life looks like. As my children have grown up and tried to find their way in the world, my encouragement to them has always been to find their passion in life and to pursue that passion, whatever it may be. There is a story of a man whose car was stuck on the train tracks at a crossing, with the train rapidly bearing down on him. As he tried to start his car, he realized he had a choice to make: try to restart his car and move it or abandon the vehicle to save his own life. He was undecided, waffling until it was too late. The reality was that the man had made a choice, whether he wanted to or not. There was a default position: the choice to remain on the track was the choice made until he decided to do something else.

The choice to follow a passion is similar: it is a choice that requires intention and effort. Anything less is default. My children know that, regardless of their choice of vocation, if they do it because they are passionate about it, I will support them to the bitter end. This, whether they choose to be teachers, mechanics, neurosurgeons, or musicians.

We all have the choice to live intentionally and contentedly in our circumstances, good or bad. This choice, *vive ut vivas,* is above all a deliberate one; living "so that you may live" will never just happen on its own.

I have learned that obsessing about things I cannot change does not do me any good and is ultimately self-defeating.
Trying to change things that I cannot change causes me to miss the joy in the things that I can do and can change. In his wonderful one-man play, *This Is Cancer,* Bruce Horak quotes his own father

when he says, "'Cancer gave me something. It gave me time.'" Time to live. While on the surface the idea that a terminal disease would be credited with providing time to live seems crazy, it often does that very thing. It provides the clarity to recognize how important it is to repair a relationship, watch a sunset, plant a tree, and remember what loving the people around you really means. It is sad that we so often wait until the end to address such matters, when our days could be made easier to bear if we attended to the critical things sooner. We need to spend more time laughing, crying, and looking hopefully to the future and to spend less time worrying about things, people, and relationships beyond our control.

I have learned that we all have an expiry date, but this date is never stamped on our birth certificate.

This is not meant to be flippant about life and death; I recognize full well that some people who read this will be grappling with their own imminent death or the death of someone close to them. However, no one is immortal. Whether you get cancer or not, you are going to die. Beat cancer or not, you are going to die. To vary the old adage, death is the only guarantee in life—because some people do manage to avoid taxes.

I have learned that when my life comes to a close, only two things are left: to love those whom I must let go, and allow myself to be released by those who love me.

My friend Reg fought for his life. But there came a certain point when his family was able to sit with him and release him from the further exhaustion of struggle into the inevitable result of his disease. And with that, he was able to release his life into the hands of God; shortly thereafter he was dead. His wife and daughters wept over him, but they did not beg him to hang on for just one more day. And he, while never desiring to hasten his own death, recognized that his life, being the gift of grace, had never really belonged to him in the first place, and that he had no right to clutch onto it as though it were his by right.

Finally, I have learned that sometimes a short time lived with quality and dignity is better than a prolonged time of suffering and anguish.

This one is hard. While I am not a proponent of assisted suicide and, in fact, would say that I am in the "firmly opposed" camp, I think there are times to hang on to life and times to let go. There are times to fight and times to give in. And there are times for heroic measures and times for choosing quality over quantity. As a result, it is important that you talk to your friends and family about how you want your days lived. In many cases, this may involve a living will, designed in times of joy and lucidity to describe what happens when you are unable to make decisions for yourself. While I do not think it is the place of doctors to intentionally shorten the length of our days, neither is it their place to artificially lengthen those days beyond the point that we and those we love desire. I am a proud Canadian, and one of the significant contributions my country has made to the world is the development of palliative medicine, designed to bring as much kindness as possible into our final days in our bodies.

For all of us, there will be an end. And when that end comes, rarely is it welcomed. But the measure of our lives is not the length of our days; it is the quality of life lived in those days. Get cancer or not, beat cancer or not, we all have to go sometime. Cancer has taught me to hold life as precious and to make the most of the time that I have.

A Tale of Two Doctors: A Message to Health Care Providers

It was the best of times, it was the worst of times, it was the age of reason,
it was the age of foolishness, it was the epoch of belief, it was the epoch of
incredulity, it was the season of Light, it was the season of Darkness, it was
the spring of hope, it was the winter of despair, we had everything before us,
we had nothing before us, we were all going direct to Heaven, we were all
going direct the other way—in short, the period was so far like the present
period, that some of its noisiest authorities insisted on its being received, for
good or for evil, in the superlative degree of comparison only.

Charles Dickens, *A Tale of Two Cities*

In the recesses of our minds, most of us can remember deciding to be
what we have become—choosing that idealized version of our vocation.
Perhaps you can recall the moment when you realized you would be
a doctor, a nurse, a surgeon, or an oncologist. You chose to pursue an
ideal, and your choice was a good and worthy one.

But my story, my experience with practitioners of medicine, is one
rife with contrast: the good and the bad. That contrast is best conveyed
"in the superlative degree of comparison only," so I shall try to tell that
story here. My goal is not to shame or make feel guilty any health care
professional reading this. Nor are my words designed to make anyone
feel superior. My intent is simply to recount the patient's experience,
and in so doing, to affirm those parts of your practice that patients love,
and, at the same time, to challenge those parts they dread or dislike. I
am only one voice, but in my voice echo the voices of others. I do not
presume to speak for every patient, nor do I presume to assert that mine
is the only message. What I can do, however, is tell you what I think:
send my message into the wind and hope that the whisper will be loud
enough for some to hear and that its message will mean something
to the hearers.

In Part I of this book, I tried to steer away from any conclusions. While I do have definite opinions about the treatments my doctors prescribed and the attitudes they displayed towards me, I tried to let my narrative speak for itself, so that my readers could arrive at their own conclusions about who the heroes and villains in my story were. I did that primarily because I did not want to label, even privately, never mind publicly, any doctor who treated me as a "bad doctor," which I believe to be untrue and fundamentally unfair. However, here I want to be more direct and, in my own voice, presume to give my opinions, the opinions I would give were I fortunate enough to sit across a table from you and talk about my experience.

With that in mind, here are some things I've learned that I would like from my health care providers.

Tell me what you think is wrong with me, especially if I press you.

While I can recognize the value of not worrying a patient more than is necessary, especially when the diagnosis of a serious illness is unlikely, I found I was far more worried when I sensed or knew something was wrong but no one would talk to me about it than when I knew what the all possible outcomes could be.

The doctor I went to at my first walk-in clinic told me, "You have a mass on your intestine." A statement which was delivered in the same way as, "I'm having a burrito for lunch." He did not say it without empathy because I'm sure he knew what it could have been and, as a result, knew the possible implications. But he did not tell me; I suppose he wanted to leave the bad news, should it be confirmed, to come from the doctor who could fix me. When I asked what it could be, the doctor was evasive. However, I wanted—no, needed—to know what I was up against and what the spectrum of my concern should be. Nevertheless, the doctor would not let me in on the secret, as though his deferral, "We'll let the specialist take care of that," was a reassuring remark.

Remember that I am a person with feelings and that professional detachment is not always the most appropriate response to me and my illness.

My first surgeon told me, "You have cancer, and I know how to treat it. You have colorectal cancer, and you are going to need a colostomy. You have cancer, and the treatment will inflict enough damage to leave you impotent. You have cancer, and, if you need to cry, you can. You have cancer; have a nice day, and please, do come again."

Of course, he was probably not cold, callous, and unfeeling, but that is how he came across to me, sitting at one end of a large, dark room with a huge table between us.

I guess I should thank that surgeon for having had such a lousy bedside manner because it was not his diagnosis, but rather his calculated and emotionless delivery, which created in me a sense of distrust, the belief that somehow there was more information I needed to seek out. I did not let him follow through with his proposed treatment because I believed his judgement to be in line with his empathy and delivery. And, in retrospect, I was right. I am told he was a "buffoon"—this word coming from a surgeon I know—not only because of his bedside manner, but also because of his treatment plan. Given that I had a tumour only 10 centimetres into my rectum, there was no reason to plan for a colostomy.

My mother also had a surgeon, who told her she would need a hysterectomy because she had a tumour in her uterus. When my mother cried, reeling with utter shock, dismay, and fear, this doctor provided no emotional support. Instead, he implored her, "Get it together! Do you think you will grow a beard because I remove your uterus? This happens to women all the time." He failed in his duty to her.

Treat me as an intelligent person and engage me with respect as I struggle with the choices that you put before me.

An oncologist told me that I needed chemotherapy. When I replied, not with the expected gratitude and compliance, but with earnest, respectful questions arising out of documents and peer-reviewed articles (from the *New England Journal of Medicine* among others, no less), along with a request to be heard and have my questions engaged, I was met with, "Not clinically relevant," and "What is the point?" When I asked where the centres of excellence were for my disease, he did not know. When I found one next door in Ontario, he dismissed their research. He told me that if I started chemo and then stopped, I would not be able to start again, presumably a tactic designed to convince me his was the best route to take. After all, he was the expert.

Every interaction with this doctor was extremely intimidating and distressing; every meeting was anticipated with increasing anxiety and trepidation. Even after I had stopped taking chemotherapy, I went to my next appointment with him but admitted nothing, fearing I would get a stern talking-to about the reckless decision I'd made without his approval. And, upon his seeing my anxiety over the question of chemotherapy, anxiety that was the product of an honest struggle with the science around my genetics, he proclaimed he was judging me unfit to continue with chemotherapy, and he removed that option from my treatment regimen.

When you are wrong, admit it.

I know this one is hard, especially because there can be legal liability issues involved. Nevertheless, there are many circumstances that fall between the poles of being absolutely right and having performed malpractice. A patient's confidence and sense of well-being can be greatly enhanced simply by knowing that her doctor is willing to admit to fallibility. In retrospect, I realize my oncologist never once admitted he'd been wrong, said my research was probative, or acknowledged my questions as legitimate, despite their validation by experts in the field.

A few years later, another oncologist prematurely, and within easy earshot of my young teen-aged son who was terrified he might have cancer, announced a diagnosis of malignancy purportedly confirmed by pathology results, in complete contradiction to both the pathological evidence and the firm diagnosis of a surgeon his senior in age, practice, and wisdom. By now sadly accustomed to the way of careless or callous physicians, I dismissed his assessment outright as erroneous, upon which he turned heel and left, never to return. He never came back to apologize either to me or to my son. In fact, neither this oncologist nor his supervising senior doctor ever spoke to me again, not even to inform me, officially, of what I already knew—but which they had emphatically countered: that my son didn't, in fact, have cancer. Neither this oncologist, nor any supervisor of his, ever again checked on my son to query his emotional or physical well-being subsequent to the false pronouncement of malignancy, not even to ensure he understood that in fact he did not have cancer. That was left to someone else.

Some of my experience, and many things beyond my personal experience and comprehension, represent the worst of medicine. And I know that it is very rare for doctors to be called to account for any of the things they do that could easily be classified as insensitive or even bullying and cruel. Nor are they typically assessed in their practice, diagnosis, or empathy. They are never asked to sit before a patient to apologize for their actions or attitudes or to explain egregious mistakes.

Put me before your procedures, your practices, and your ego.

Dr. Pfeifer gave me a second, radically different opinion when the first doctor's diagnosis and prognosis left me confused and afraid. He didn't rashly promise, "You won't have to have a colostomy," but he did hold out that possibility only as the second-best option, the fall-back position. He said, "This is what I plan to do because it's best for you in the long run, but if that doesn't work out, we'll do the colostomy." He didn't begin his sentences with, "I am," or "You have," but, "You *are*." He acknowledged that what was to be done had naught to do with who he was as a doctor, nor was it an offensive he launched at a target disease; his treatment was service he rendered to me as a person.

Dr. Yaffe gladly provided me with a referral to an out-of-province doctor whom I believed to be the expert in my condition. He did this not just because it was his obligation, medically, to do so, but also because he knew that it would be good for me. It would calm my worry and reinforce the decisions I had made. And it would provide resources for my family and me in dealing with a permanent condition.

Dr. Lum Min sat with my wife and me as we talked about our youngest son. She did not flinch once when we asked to call in cancer experts from Toronto. She did not balk when we asked if a more experienced surgeon could assist her on the surgery that my son might need. She went out of her way on more than one occasion to reassure us that his health and healing and our efforts towards that outcome were far more important than her ego.

Remember that I am not my disease.

Dr. Pfeifer answered my call in the operating room and never once made me feel that I was intrusive or out of line in having questions.

Dr. Kyeremateng scheduled me for a CT scan when I was having abdominal pain because she knew my history and felt more concerned than I did about what might be happening in my digestive system. Her intuition ensured that my second tumour (an *interval* cancer that developed between surveillance tests) got caught eight months sooner than it would otherwise have been had I waited for my next regularly scheduled scope.

Dr. Yaffe let me waffle when I worried about the effect of a colectomy on my quality of life and the pace of my healing. He let me make appointments to talk about its implications despite the fact there was no additional information to be had.

Dr. Yaffe walked into the operating theatre where I was awaiting surgery, and, with a calming assurance, put all my fears to rest.

Dr. Yaffe stopped me in the hallway during a difficult recuperation, touched my shoulder, and told me that everything would be okay. He offered reassurance that was born out of his understanding of me and of what I needed at that moment.

A doctor's practice of medicine should be marked by competence, confidence, empathy, and humility.

Because I am not a doctor, I am not sure what gets taught in medical school. I have never been through the rigours of the process and cannot begin to comprehend the pressures that come with the education and practice of medicine. Nevertheless, that does not change what I expect as a patient, which can be summarized in four qualities that I, speaking for the collective patient, have the right to demand of all of my doctors: competence, confidence, empathy, and humility.

Doctors need to be competent. I would expect no less than that from anyone into whose hands I placed my health and my life. And that means not only the skills and knowledge that come from years in medical school, but also the ongoing training that represents a desire to give the very best to the patient.

Doctors need to be confident. They need to be able to approach my health and wholeness from the position of knowing what is right to do and how to best execute that.

Doctors need to be empathetic. The competence and confidence doctors have need to reside firmly within an empathetic attitude. The one that sees me as a whole person and not as a tumour to be resected nor a disease to be cured. I am a father, a husband, a worker, a student, a brother, a son. I am so much more than my disease, and whatever is done to me or with me has to take my whole life into account. Patient history is not just about medical facts.

Finally, doctors need to be humble. This humility does not conflict with either competence or confidence. It recognizes one's personal limitations alongside the ability of others, even the weak and uneducated, to speak into situations. It recognizes that insight may come from many angles and sources. Humility recognizes that it's the doctor's responsibility to acknowledge that potential for insight. Humility does not require that every whim of the patient be humoured, but it does require that the patient be taken seriously and listened to respectfully. Sometimes, if you listen with an attuned ear, you can be surprised at what you hear.

Of course, these four things—competence, confidence, empathy, and humility—apply not just to doctors, but to all medical personnel and to people in all areas of human interaction. However, it seems that the high status of a physician has too much of a tendency to relegate these qualities to the background and replace them with a spirit of competition and arrogance. It requires strength of will and the grit of determination to allow what is good to predominate; becoming and remaining an excellent professional is never an easy thing.

Part 3

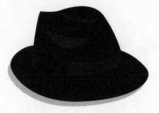

Conversations
with a Doctor

Writing, when properly managed (as you may be sure I think mine is) is but a different name for conversation.

Laurence Sterne,
The Life and Times of Tristram Shandy, Gentleman

-35-

We Talk About Cancer

As in the experimental sciences, truth cannot be distinguished from error as long as firm principles have not been established through the rigorous observation of facts.

Louis Pasteur, *Études sur la maladie des vers à soie*

"A guy walks into his doctor's office ... ." That could be the start of a bad joke or a great conversation, so I chose the latter. Here is how it went.

I sat in my doctor's waiting room, the kind that looked as though it had been decorated in the 1950s, with orange chairs and tables made of wood that would be illegal to use had they been made today.

"Dennis." I heard his receptionist call my name. "Just step in here, and the doctor will be right with you."

I took a seat in the small room and grabbed the complimentary 1995 issue of *Reader's Digest* from the stand. I flipped to "Drama in Real Life." I always love that. It was about a guy who gets caught in the desert and has to chase down and eat a camel to survive. A harrowing tale.

"Dennis! Great to see you. How are you?"

"I'm well, thanks."

"How can I help you today?"

"I want you to tell me about cancer, doc."

"What do you want to know?"

I began, "I was reading on *Wikipedia* the other day—"

"Wait, wait. That's your first mistake, Dennis."

"What?"

"Your first mistake is going to *Wikipedia* for your information about cancer."

"Where should I go?"

"Well, I'd start here, with me. If you want Internet information, look at the web sites of cancer societies, hospitals, and cancer clinics."

"Okay. Well, here I am. Can I ask you some questions?"

"Sure, you're my last patient of the day; ask away."

"Cancer seems to be everywhere, but there are so many kinds. How would you describe what it is?"

"Well, Dennis, cancer is not so much a thing as a collection of things. There are hundreds of diseases that we've come to call cancer, and they have only a few things in common."

"What are they?"

"Fundamentally, cancer is a collection of bad cells that refuse to die. You see, your body is always producing new cells, and in the process, it's actually not uncommon for slight irregularities to form in the DNA of a cell. Whenever that happens there is first a process by which the body attempts to repair the error. If that does not work, there's a kill switch the body will normally flip so as to get rid of that cell. If the irregular cell then dies off, it can't reproduce, and the problem is dealt with. However, sometimes your body misses the problem, can't fix it, or the kill switch is defective, and that cell lives to reproduce. If the cell cluster gets to be between 16 and 64 cells big—about four to six generations old—we call it *malignant* or cancerous, and you have a problem."

"So, that process is the only thing all these diseases have in common? Then why just one name?"

"That generic, lay term fits the general category of this host of diseases. Moreover, we have always used this general term, and it would cause a lot of confusion if we suddenly started calling these diseases by different names. Can you imagine the result if someone came to your door trying to raise money for research into *ductal carcinoma in situ* and *invasive lobular carcinoma*? Yet those names represent two kinds of breast cancer, a cause to which funds are donated every single day. Or imagine people's confused looks over requests to support efforts against *malignant melanoma, Kaposi's sarcoma,* and *cutaneous T-cell lymphoma*—all of which are kinds of skin cancer.

"Besides, ever since the Greek physician, Hippocrates, father of modern medicine, recorded the presence of what he called *carcinoma*—a Greek word meaning *crab,* which the Roman physician Celcus later translated into Latin as *cancer*—we've been stuck with the name."

"Hippocrates? I thought cancer was a new thing."

"Cancer has apparently been around since the beginning of life on earth. Recent discoveries have shown what appear to be cancer cells in the fossils of dinosaurs, so we can be confident that this isn't a new disease and that we, as humans, are not responsible for having caused it—although we continue to engage in ridiculous practices that make it much more common that it needs to be. From a human history perspective, we can find references to it as far back as ancient Egypt, where it was described as 'having no treatment.' Hippocrates used the word for a crab, *carcinoma,* to refer to certain kinds of tumours, presumably because the tumours he observed had projections growing into the surrounding tissue, bringing to mind the shape of a crab."

"So has cancer always been treated the same way?"

"No, and for two reasons. First, in ancient days, they had no idea what cancer was, and there was wild postulation about what caused it. You can imagine what kinds of treatments resulted from the idea that cancer was "an excess of black bile," for example. Second, they lacked the technology to treat it in any meaningful way other than surgical removal, which was a problem in itself, especially in the days before anaesthetics and the understanding of sterilization and infection. It was not until the middle of the 20th century that we started experimenting with radiation and chemicals as additional ways to treat cancer."

"So what about words like *lymphoma, melanoma*, and *blastoma*?"

"There are countless words used when we talk about cancers, and those are just some of them. However, it's easier to talk about a cancer when you can isolate it within a specific group, so you'll hear doctors talk about five groups of cancers: carcinomas, sarcomas, leukaemia, lymphoma and myeloma, and central nervous system cancers."

"What do those words mean?"

"Here is the brief version," he said, as he began to count off on his fingers. "One, carcinomas arise in the tissues in and around organs and include colon cancer, skin cancer, lung cancer, liver cancer, and a whole bunch of other cancers that form as solid tumours. Two, sarcomas arise in supportive tissues such as bones and cartilage. Three, leukaemias are cancers in the areas of the body that make blood, such as bone marrow; too often, these cancers are borne by children. Four, lymphomas and myelomas are cancers which arise in the cells forming the immune system, specifically the lymph system. And finally, central nervous system cancers arise in the brain and spinal column."

"Are these cancers all detected and treated the same way?"

"No. Because each group is rather unique, they generally have their own method of detection and treatment. But even within a group, such as carcinomas, some organs are easier to detect cancer in than others. For example, you can get a carcinoma in your colon, which can be detected with a colonoscope that can also grab tissue at the same time for testing in the lab. Or you can get a carcinoma in your pancreas, which is generally detected with a CT scan before being confirmed by separate biopsy procedure. Colonoscopies are relatively routine procedures, whereas pancreatic biopsies are not. This is one of the many reasons that colon cancers are more often detected early, allowing treatment to begin early, whereas pancreatic cancers are often detected too late for effective treatment."

"I suppose treatments are limited by the kind of cancer as well. Obviously you can't have surgery to remove cancer in your blood."

"That's right. You can't remove cancer in your blood by cutting it out. Instead, a combination of radiation and chemotherapy is done to rid the body of that cancer."

"But, I'm pretty sure—even with solid tumours that surgery can cut out—the cancer does not always stay where it started. I heard of a guy who supposedly had testicular cancer, but they found it in his brain. They said it had spread there."

"Yes, it would have *metastasized*. That means it had moved from one place to another. Sometimes this movement is from one organ to an adjacent one. So, for example, if you have colon cancer, that cancer can grow out of the colon and into the liver or kidneys—anything the colon touches. In addition, because we have the blood and lymph systems that move material throughout the body, it's also possible for cancer cells to break off, travel throughout the body, and begin to grow new tumours wherever they land. Those new tumours would still be considered to be the same kind of cancer that the defective cells were to begin with. So, you can end up with a colon tumour in the liver or a testicular tumour in the brain."

"That sounds really scary."

"Yes, it is. Metastatic cancer can be very dangerous and is too often fatal. However, it's not always a death sentence because treatment options have come a long way, and many people recover from even advanced metastatic cancer."

"I have a friend who had cancer, and his doctor gave it a number, which also had something to do with how advanced it was, I think."

"Yes, most cancers have different standard identification schemes to allow doctors to gauge how advanced and serious the disease is. In the past, there were various numbering and lettering patterns, but these days they use a three-part system to try to identify the severity. In solid tumours, this system gauges the localization of the tumour, the involvement of lymph nodes, and the distance of the tumour from the original site, or whether it has metastasized."

"Whoa, doc, can we take these things one at a time? Localization?"

"Localization is basically an indication of how large the tumour is, how much it has progressed into the organ where it began, and how much it's impacting the organs in direct proximity to the original site. A tumour which forms on the inside of the colon and hasn't progressed out of the colon would be characterized as a localized tumour. If it has moved outside of the colon and into adjacent organs, it would no longer be localized."

"So a tumour that's localized would be easier to treat than one that isn't, right?"

"That's right."

"Okay. So what is lymph node involvement?"

"Lymph node involvement is determined both by imaging, using MRI or CT scan, and by dissecting lymph nodes in the tumour tissue removed by a surgeon. The lymph system is a series of interconnected nodes that collect and filter waste fluids from your body. Because this system pervades the body, it has the unfortunate ability to transport cancer cells everywhere should it be infiltrated. Therefore, the amount of invasion into your lymph nodes is an important indicator of the severity and progress of a cancer. The greater the number of lymph nodes involved, the greater the risk potential of the cancer."

"So, if there's lymph node involvement, it's possible that cells from the tumour will have moved into other parts of the body?"

"Again, right."

"What about distance of cancer from the original site? Isn't that simply the idea of localization again?"

"Well, yes and no. Localization is strictly about tumour size and growth at the original site, whereas distance from the original site is about the tumour transplanting itself into a distant organ—such as testicular cancer showing up in your brain. Cells from any tumour which is found can be examined to determine what kind of cells they are. Because each organ and its cancer is unique—liver cancer cells look different from lung cancer cells—an analysis of a tumour can often indicate where those cells originated. Metastatic cancer of any kind is the most serious because it means that cancer cells are moving into distant organs and that more radical treatment methods are likely required."

"So, once you have these three things measured, what's next?"

"These characteristics are then blended together to determine the overall stage. This works as a kind of short cut, bypassing the minutia and getting to the heart of the matter: how serious the cancer is. A number–letter combination is used to describe or *stage* a cancer, which is useful in providing a good estimate as to how serious it is and how aggressive the treatment will need to be. In addition, the stage provides an indication of the *prognosis*, that is, what the chances of survival for a given period of time are. It may seem self-evident, but, the lower the stage, the better the average cure rate is and the greater the chance of being alive five years later."

"Okay, wait. I've heard this before: *prognosis* and *five-year survival rate*. What's up with that? When my uncle had cancer, there was no talk of his dying, ever, and yet the doctor insisted on talking about the five-year survival rate. It really freaked him out!"

"Yes, I wish there were a better way to express that, but this is really statistics talking. First of all, your prognosis is what the doctor thinks is going to happen to you. While diagnosis is the identification of what you have, prognosis is the best guess as to whether you are going to get better, how quickly, and at what cost. The doctor may talk generally about prognosis when she says, 'The prognosis is usually good for tumours of this sort.' In that case, she's talking about the overall treatability of a certain kind of cancer. However, patients are typically more interested in their individual prognosis than a general one."

"Okay, but what about this five-year survival rate? Sounds rather grim."

"It sounds grim, yes, but again, note that it's statistics talking when we tell you about five-year survival rates; these numbers apply to large populations. For example, when you flip a coin, the likelihood of getting heads is 50%. Yet sometimes you can flip three heads in a row, completely against the odds. Once you've flipped the coin 1,000 or 10,000 times, however, you are going to see results which are very close to a 50% heads rate: that is the reality which statistics describe. So, we talk about five-year survival rates because statisticians look at a large sample of patients, group them together based on the characteristics of their disease, and then identify the likelihood of their getting better."

"But why five years? Isn't that an arbitrary time frame?"

"Yes, but you need to pick some time period. The thing about five years is, first, there are a lot of data for that, so you can easily come up with the statistics. Second, five years is a short enough period to reduce the chance of other illnesses or accidents getting in the way of accurately assessing the effects of cancer on mortality. Look at an alternative: let's say that you talked about a 25-year survival rate. Well, we know that there would be significantly fewer people alive 25 years after being diagnosed with cancer than five years after, but there would be no practical way to know how many of those people had died from an accident or disease other than cancer, so a survival rate with that long a time frame would hold no useful information. The time frame to measure survival is reduced to five years in order to isolate the effect of one specific disease, in this case, cancer, on mortality."

"So if my doctor talks about five-year survival, that has nothing to do with him worrying about my being around in five years?"

"Not at all. It's just a way to talk about the efficacy of current treatment methods. Also note that as treatments are improving, the five-year survival rate is also getting better, even though you won't see it reflected in the statistics right away. If a radically better treatment for something shows up tomorrow, it's going to take a while before the five-year survival rate has incorporated the greater numbers of people surviving."

"So, how is cancer treated?"

"Despite many advancements in specific therapies, there are really only three basic ways to treat cancer: with chemicals (chemotherapy), radiation, and surgery."

"How do these treatments work?"

"Well, surgery is pretty straightforward, at least as a concept, if not in its execution. The surgeon identifies something that shouldn't be a part of you and removes it by cutting it out. She intends to accomplish a few goals in the process. The first is to excise the entire tumour while removing as little of the surrounding tissue as possible. During surgery, an attempt is made to get the whole tumour while ensuring *clear margins.*"

"Clear margins?"

"That means a reasonable amount of healthy tissue around the tumour. If you get all of the tumour out, and the margins are clear, you have not left any cancer behind, at least none that can be detected in the operating theatre or the lab."

"I see."

"Surgery has a second goal: to preserve function. That means the surgeon intends the body to function the same after the surgery as it did beforehand. Now, this isn't always possible, but it's the goal that the surgeon strives for. Sometimes this is straightforward. However, sometimes it becomes a balancing act between these two goals. It may be that a reduction in function is required in order to get clear margins.

On the other hand, it may be that clear margins are not possible while still preserving the life of the patient, which you can appreciate easily happens with brain surgery, for example. In those cases, a compromise would have to be reached while looking towards a second surgery or some other treatment after recovery to get the best possible result."

"So, two goals for surgery then?"

"No, there's a third goal, a diagnostic one. Generally, tissue is extracted for testing. For example, lymph nodes around the site of the tumour are extracted for the purpose of testing them for malignant cells. This is used diagnostically to help determine the spread and severity of the cancer."

"But not all·cancers can be treated surgically, right?"

"That's correct. Some, such as leukaemia, can't be treated surgically at all because the individual cancer cells are distributed throughout the body. Other cases of cancer might be too advanced for complete treatment through surgery: cancer cells may have progressed beyond the original tumour into the blood or lymph, or even from there to new tumour sites. In those cases, alternative or additional treatments are necessary."

"So, that would mean chemo or radiation then, right?"

"Yes, one or both of those."

"So, sometimes more than one treatment is used for a cancer?"

"Yes. In fact, that happens frequently, and in some cases, all three are used. Surgery is used when there's a solid tumour that can be located and removed. However, sometimes the surgery needs to be preceded by chemo or radiation or both to shrink the tumour first. In other cases, chemo or radiation, or a combination of both, is used to get rid of cancer that might remain after surgery."

"I understand how surgery works: you cut things out. How do chemotherapy and radiation work?"

"These are two different processes. Let me tackle radiation first. Radiation is very dangerous, in general, whether it comes from nuclear power or naturally in the form of radon gas in your home. Exposure to radiation has certainly been responsible for many cancer diagnoses. While it may seem counter-intuitive, that danger is actually connected to the same reason radiation is effective against cancer. When any cell, cancerous or not, is exposed to radiation, the DNA can get messed up and stop reproducing. That's the principle behind radiation therapy. A beam of particles is aimed at the site of the cancer with the intent of killing off the cancer cells. This can be quite an effective treatment over time. However, it's not without its own risks. Because you're exposing both the cancerous and the healthy tissues to radiation, you run the risk of messing up the DNA of healthy cells, so that they run riot in reproducing and become cancerous too. Some studies have shown that women who were given radiation therapy for breast cancer when they were young have a greater chance of developing other cancers in their chests as they age."

"So, they target radiation at patients with some kind of a ray gun?"

"Well, this is not Buck Rogers, so it's delivered with a large machine, not a hand-held gun, but, essentially, yes. For some forms of cancer, however, they have created more effective radiation delivery systems. A current treatment for prostate cancer has a surgeon implant a set of radioactive seeds into a patient using a series of needles. This has the advantage of being a continuous delivery system, and the source of radiation is in close proximity to the tumour."

"What about chemotherapy?"

"Chemotherapy, or *chemo*, as it is typically known, uses chemicals to kill cancer cells. The chemicals can be put into the body either by swallowing pills or being injected as an intravenous solution. Regardless of the delivery system, the basic premise is the same: find the cells in the body that are reproducing rapidly and kill them."

"So, chemotherapy targets the cancer cells?"

"Not specifically. What it's looking for are cells that are dividing rapidly, a characteristic of cancer cells. However, cancer cells are not the only kind of cells in our bodies that divide rapidly, so by killing these other fast-growing cells, chemo can cause side effects."

"You mean hair loss and nausea?"

"Yes. Some cells in the body naturally reproduce rapidly. These would include blood cells, hair follicles, and the cells that line the digestive system. Because these cells are also damaged by chemo, there's the chance that hair will fall out, you'll experience anaemia and weakness, and you'll have digestive problems such as nausea, sometimes very intensely. However, there are treatments that can be used to alleviate some of these symptoms, and because *oncologists*—specialists in cancer—are getting better at regulating dosages for certain cancers, many of these side effects are milder than they would have been even a decade ago."

"So, chemo is used to remove tumours or shrink them before surgery."

"Yes, but not just that. Chemo is used for five things. First, it can sometimes be *curative*; that is, it can completely rid the body of cancer, as in blood-borne cancers such as leukaemia. Second, it can be used as an *adjuvant therapy*. That means it's used after another primary treatment, following surgery, for example, in order to rid the body of cancer cells that can't be removed by surgery or can't be seen, yet are suspected to be present."

"So adjuvant chemotherapy sometimes ends up being used even when there's no cancer at all, just because of a suspicion?"

"Yes, sometimes adjuvant therapy is prescribed as a precaution against cancer that might be present but can't actually be detected."

"You said there were five uses for chemo. What are the other three?"

"The third use is called *neoadjuvant therapy*. That's chemo administered before the primary treatment, usually in an attempt to shrink the tumour in preparation for surgery. The fourth use is *palliative*. This is done when cancer can't be removed from the body: the objective is to extend patients' lives and to improve their quality of life by either shrinking or slowing down the growth of a cancer so that its symptoms are reduced. Palliative treatment is not focused on saving the patient's life but on extending it and maximizing the patient's level of comfort."

"And the fifth use?"

"Yes, there is one more, but technically it doesn't belong to the treatment category because it's preventative. This is a new field, and it doesn't look at chemotherapy in the conventional way. In reality, any chemical treatment for cancer is chemotherapy, and these days, there has been a lot of research into the effectiveness of that common but mysterious drug, Aspirin, against many diseases, including cancer. Promising research shows that, in some people, relatively large doses of Aspirin are effective in preventing some kinds of tumours from forming on the intestinal wall. And, of course, the hope is that one day we'll find drugs that will prevent all kinds of cancers."

"So, if scientists are doing research into specific drugs that will prevent cancer, we must know what causes it."

"Well, not really; not yet, anyway. We've identified some pretty strong contributors to the formation of cancer, but there are very few one-to-one causal factors we know about."

"What about smoking? Haven't we determined that smoking causes lung cancer?"

"While it's true smoking is very bad for people and contributes to serious health problems, its relationship with the disease is not directly causal, even with lung cancer. Let me give you an example before I explain. If you take a gun and shoot your foot, it will do damage. And every time you shoot your foot under the same conditions, you'll do the same damage. That is direct causation: the gunshot causes the damage. However, not everyone exposed to *carcinogenic* or cancer-causing substances such as chemicals in cigarette smoke or asbestos gets cancer. You might be surprised, for example, to know that while smoking is the primary cause of all lung cancers, only 10–20% of people who smoke end up with lung cancer. That's not to say that smoking is benign, because it contributes to a whole host of health problems, including emphysema and heart disease. Nevertheless, there is no direct path between smoking and lung cancer; it's more complex than that."

"So there are other contributing factors that make cancer more likely for one person and less likely for the next?"

"Yes. Those factors include diet, exercise, environmental hazards, genetics, and even previous diseases. For example, in the 1950s, it was not uncommon for children of farmers to act as helpers during pesticide spraying. My mother tells stories of coming home covered in DDT because she'd stand at the end of a crop row with a flag to help her dad spray a straight row, and she'd get covered with chemicals as he pulled the tractor around her. It's very possible, and probable, perhaps, that her exposure to these chemicals may contribute to cancer at some point in her lifetime."

"How do genetics play a part in cancer? I know people who have family trees full of relatives who've had cancer. Can I get cancer from my parents?"

"Well, that's going to take a bit more explaining. I'll tell you what: why don't you stop by next week, and we can talk about genetics and cancer then, okay?"

"Sure, doc. That was helpful. See you in a week, same time?"

"Same time."

I left his office with a head full of facts, understanding a lot more and ready to try committing it all to my notebook.

36

We Talk About Genetics
and Cancer

We will now discuss in a little more detail the struggle for existence.

Charles Darwin, *On the Origin of the Species*

I returned to my doctor's office the following week with more questions.

I opened, "So, doc, we left off at the topic of cancer and genetics. Does cancer have a genetic component, and, if so, can I get cancer from my parents?"

"That's a complicated question. In general, the answer is no, but sometimes the answer is yes, and that depends both on what your question is actually asking and what kind of cancer you are talking about. While some cancers actually come about as the result of genetic mutations passed from parent to child, most of the time the process is more complicated and nuanced than that. But, let's back up a bit first, and then take a running start at the topic of cancer and genetics, okay?"

"Review? Sounds good to me."

"So, I think that we left off talking about how different people, exposed to the same environments, do not always react the same way. Furthermore, one person will get cancer where another will not, due to a combination of factors such as stress levels, age, other illnesses, diet, exercise, sleep, and genetics."

"So far so good. Now, you've already talked about the central role of genes—in terms of messed-up DNA—in how cancer starts in people. Usually, though, it's hereditary issues I think of when I hear the word *genetics.*"

"What I'd explained was that cancer happens when subtle problems arise in the replication of DNA as a cell reproduces. Normally, the body detects this error and fixes the problem or kills the broken cells. When these flaws are not caught, however, but are replicated over and over again, eventually they cannot be stopped by the body's natural systems, and they become cancer. In that sense, all cancer is genetic. However, when most people talk about genetics, you're right, they mean traits that pass from parent to child, and some of these traits can contribute to your body being able or unable, as the case may be, to fight cancer as it is arising."

"You say *contribute*. So, then, I don't get some sort of cancer gene from my parents?"

"Generally not. Most cancer syndromes don't cause cancer, not per se. What usually happens is that genetic characteristics might allow one person to fight cancer as it is forming or to react to a harmful environment better than another person. Genetic weaknesses can also be passed on: things that make one person less able than another to fight a developing cancer and therefore more likely to get it."

"How do I get genetic characteristics, and what are these?"

"Hmm, I think I need to summarize Genetics 101 for you. Ready?"

"Okay, let me have it."

"Genetics is the basis of life, all life. It's the fundamental building block of reproduction and the differentiation of species. And despite the fact that my genes are 99.9% the same as yours and between 96% and 98% the same as a chimp's, I am neither you nor a chimp. My DNA defines who I am—or at least what my potential is—when I'm born. Genes, sometimes called chromosomes, define the colour of my skin, eyes, and hair. They define the potential range of my height, weight, and IQ. These genes are contained inside a twisted ladder called deoxyribonucleic acid—DNA—which is contained within all the cells in my body."

"DNA is a twisted ladder?"

"DNA is a protein which defines your full genetic make-up. It's the foundation of life, and, once established at the point of your conception, is fundamentally unchangeable. Your DNA defines all things biological about you. Typically, it's described as a double helix, that is, a ladder shape which has been twisted to look like a set of circular stairs. Half of your DNA template comes from your biological mother through her egg and the other half from your biological father through his sperm."

"So, we have these little ladders in our cells?"

"In essence, yes. And the structure consists of 23 groupings, called chromosomes, which are connected in pairs by chemicals, and which look like the rungs of a ladder. You get half of your chromosomes from your mother and half from your father. People whose genetics deviate from this standard 23-pair template tend to have physical and mental disabilities as compared to the average population. For example, people with Down syndrome have an extra copy of chromosome 21—rather than two of chromosomes, they have three. This defect manifests itself in physical and mental impairment, to a greater or lesser extent from individual to individual."

"Let's see. DNA is made up of chromosomes, and I have 23 paired sets?"

"Right. Now, a gene is a piece of a chromosome: every human cell has about 25,000 genes. Scientists have determined the functions of some genes, and they've also identified common errors, or mutations, that occur in these genes, as well as what their ill effects are. Genes are responsible for your physical traits; for example, your hair colour. The particular variant of a certain gene that you have is called an *allele*, and you have two of each, one from your mother and one from your father. It is the combination of the alleles you inherited that will determine whether your hair colour is auburn, blonde, or dark brown. Think of the options available when you buy a new car. Every car has a colour (gene) and the palette of colours that can be chosen from (alleles). Once you choose from the set of possible colours, you have, fixed for all time, the colour of your new car. In a similar manner, there is a gene or allele-pair responsible for the colour of your hair. Various alleles for human hair colour options exist, but you will end up with one of your father's two hair-colour alleles and one of your mother's pair, which together will determine your hair colour. The variation between your hair colour and someone else's is due to your alleles for the same gene being different than the other person's."

"So, let me get this straight. Alleles determine characteristics, and they are grouped in *mom–pop* pairs as 25,000 genes, which are all grouped together into 23 paired chromosome sets that look like a ladder and make up the DNA which is in every cell and unique to me?"

"That's correct, unless you are an identical twin, triplet, or quadruplet, for example. In that case, the other person has the same DNA as you."

"Ending up with my mother's nose and my father's eyes is the result of their paired alleles in a gene forming a characteristic in me?"

"Yes. Some of these characteristics are simple, but most are really complex. Eye colour is relatively straightforward, so I'll use that as an example. However, before I start, I need to explain dominant and recessive."

"Haha, I know that. I've got two cats. One is dominant and the other is recessive."

"Not quite what I was going for, but it's a start. Now, this is simplified, but it will get the general idea across. Review: for each physical characteristic you have, there is a gene. And for each gene, there is a pair of alleles—one that you got from each of your parents. Now, some traits on an allele are dominant, and some are recessive. Think of it as two friends: one is loud, and the other quiet. When you are with them, you always hear the loud one even though the quiet one is there too; she is the recessive one. When will you hear the quiet one? Only when you've got two quiet friends together.

"The expression of traits works in the same fashion. A dominant allele is like a loud friend; if it's paired with a recessive allele—a quiet friend—you will be aware only of the characteristics of the dominant one because the recessive one is too quiet to be heard."

"Can you give me a specific example?"

"Yes, take eye colour, for example. Brown is a dominant colour, and blue is recessive. Because brown is dominant, someone who has brown eyes could have either a pair of brown alleles or one brown one and one blue one, since the blue one would be too quiet to be noticed. On the other hand, if someone has blue eyes, it means that two blue alleles are present, and nothing else."

"Okay, I get that. Two browns make brown, a brown and a blue make brown, and two blues make blue. Right?"

"Yes. So, a man with brown eyes and two brown alleles marries a woman with blue eyes and two blue alleles. The man's sperm are all brown because he has nothing else to give out, eye-colour wise. And the woman's eggs are all blue because all her alleles are blue. Their kids each get one brown and one blue allele, so they all have brown eyes. But they also each have one blue allele just sitting quietly in the background. Now, say one of these brown-eyed children, a daughter, falls in love with a man who also has brown eyes. Little does she know, at the time, that he has one blue and one brown allele, just as she does. Half of his sperm are blue, and half are brown. Half of her eggs are blue, and half are brown. They have four children, and all of them have brown eyes except for their youngest, a girl with bright blue eyes. Statistically speaking, chances were 25% that any child they had would have two brown alleles, 50% that a child would have one brown and one blue, and 25% that a child would have two blue alleles. And it is that one in four kids with two blue alleles who will have blue eyes. That's what happened in my family. My dad has brown eyes; my mom has blue. I have brown eyes and my wife has blue eyes. We have three kids and, against the odds, all of them have blue eyes."

"Interesting! Are we getting to cancer soon?"

"Yes. At conception, your DNA was established, as were the physical manifestations of all the alleles you have. Certain alleles produce illness—for example, Huntington's disease. Others produce illness but only under certain circumstances, as with haemophilia: women are primarily carriers, but men tend to be the ones who exhibit that disease. Finally, some alleles produce weaknesses of various types which can predispose people to illness such as cancer."

"When you say *predispose*, what does that mean?"

"Well, in cases such as Huntington's, there is no predisposition: you either have the allele and the disease, or you do not. The genes involved in these cases have specific and sure effects. However, in most of the the cancer syndromes, there is a different scenario at play. What you end up with, rather than the certain presence of the disease, is a higher than normal incidence of it. The genes don't cause cancer per se; instead, they eliminate or reduce the efficacy of certain biological processes that would normally allow your body to kill off cancer. So, while a single Huntington's allele will ensure you get Huntington's disease, a cancer syndrome allele means you're more likely—and in some cases much more likely—to get cancer, but it's not guaranteed."

"And these cancer syndrome alleles, are they recessive?"

"No, they are dominant. That means a parent with the syndrome would have one defective allele in a pair and would either pass this on to a child or not: it's a 50% chance. Any child getting the broken or mutated allele would have the syndrome and would be more susceptible to cancer."

"You say one broken allele. Can't you have two, one from each parent?"

"Yes, it's possible that both alleles in a gene pair are broken. However, in those cases, the likelihood of cancer is drastically increased, and in many cases, multiple cancers occur at a very young age, which means that most children with two defective alleles don't survive long enough to reproduce. Tragically, they often die in childhood."

"Can you give me some examples of these cancer syndromes?"

"Yes. Quite a few have been identified. Now, keep in mind that these are genetic problems, or mutations, which are passed on from parents to their children, and if you look at family trees, you can

see strong evidence of these syndromes in the many cancers that are
present. However, the cancers they allow also occur—indeed much
more often—in the general population as a result of other factors,
not genetics. So the *type* of cancer alone, say, colon cancer, cannot tell
you whether a cancer syndrome is involved. Thus, genetic tests have
been created to check for certain mutations, and if a test confirms the
presence of a syndrome, surveillance plans are established, and proactive
or preventative treatment options are discussed with the patients."

"What kinds of cancers are caused by these mutations?"

"There are many, but in the news over the last several years, three
that have been talked about are colon cancer, breast cancer, and a certain
kind of eye cancer."

"In the news?"

"Yes. And it's the ones in the news that tend to get funding as
public awareness grows. Tragically, because cancer syndromes don't
affect a large percentage of the population, their research is often not
well-funded until a popular figure brings the need into the public eye."

"For example?"

"Well, in 2013, Angelina Jolie had a double mastectomy, a
preventative surgery to reduce her chances of getting breast cancer
from about 85% down to 5%. She carries a bad gene, BRCA1, which
predisposes women like her to very high rates of breast cancer. By the
way, the average woman's chance of getting breast cancer in her lifetime
is about 12%."

"Are there other syndromes like this?"

"Yes. There are at least five different mutations collectively known
as Lynch syndrome, which predisposes people to colon and other
cancers. For this group, the chances of getting colon cancer over their
lifetime are about 80%, compared to the average of 7% for the rest of
the population."

"80%! Are there no cures for these mutations?"

"Currently, there aren't. Careful surveillance can only watch closely
for the cancers and remove and treat them once they arise. In addition,
proactive surgery can remove the organ in which the cancers commonly
occur, such as the colon or the breasts, so the tumours have less chance
of developing. But there is no cure for bad genes."

"What do you do if you have a mutation?"

"Well, identification is an important thing as it tends to make
doctors more amenable to providing regular surveillance. For example,
people with Lynch syndrome get colonoscopies every year or two from

a young age onward. This is in contrast to the rest of the population, where it's recommended you get a colonoscopy at age 50, followed by another one every ten years or so, at least in the United States. In Canada, colonoscopies are not used in the general population as a regular surveillance tool.

"In addition, there are some promising results with new drug therapies that seem to suppress the rate at which cancers develop in certain areas of the body. Aspirin, that intriguing substance, seems to have positive effects for some people, including Lynch patients, in reducing the incidence of cancer. But, that research is ongoing, so don't go out and start self-medicating."

"Wow, I had no idea that cancer was so intricate and complicated."

"That's what makes the science so fascinating and the disease so terrifying."

"Well, thanks, doc. I hope we get a chance to talk like this again."

Once more, I left his office, my head full of knowledge.

37

We Talk About Cancer Prevention

About 2 in 5 Canadians will develop cancer in their lifetime, and about 1 in 4 Canadians will die of cancer. In 2014, it is estimated that 191,300 Canadians will develop cancer [plus 76,100 who will get non-melanoma skin cancer] and 76,600 will die of cancer. More than half of new cancer cases (52%) will be lung, breast, colorectal and prostate cancer.

Health Canada/Canadian Cancer Society, *Cancer Statistics 2014*

Every year the Canadian Cancer Society, in conjunction with Health Canada, issues a document publishing statistics on cancer and outlining cancer trends in Canada. There is no reason to believe that the statistics in the United States and other developed countries should not be proportional. Given that the population of the United States is about 10 times that of Canada, for instance, almost two and three-quarters million Americans will develop cancer in 2014, and over three-quarters of a million Americans will die of it.

Shocked and confused by this revelation, I once again found myself in my doctor's office, looking for answers.

I started in, "I thought that we'd made great strides towards curing cancer, but this latest Health Canada report shocks and worries me. It seems as though we have so far to go that we can never succeed."

"From a medical and scientific perspective, we have accomplished a lot and come a long way, yes, but significant obstacles still remain."

"Do you mean sequencing DNA and looking at killing cancer stem cells—that kind of thing?" I asked, hoping to impress him with the cutting-edge cancer research I'd been reading about.

"Well, those are valid areas of inquiry, but that's not at all what I meant. I think that the biggest obstacle to people being healthy and cancer-free—well, disease-free in general—is not a lack of scientific advance."

"Really?"

"Yes. The biggest obstacle is that we've failed to make the lifestyle changes required in order to prevent disease."

"What do you mean?"

"As difficult as this is for people to accept, the fact is that much of the cancer we get is due to our lifestyle and diet, and ultimately those are in our control."

"That sounds a bit too much like a 'blame the victim' mentality. How can you say it's my fault if I get cancer?"

"I would never say it's your fault. However, when educating people and talking at a societal level, I will say emphatically that we have a lot of blame to shoulder when it comes to considering why cancer is so endemic."

"Give me an example."

"Sure—exercise! Look at this report. Dr. Dhali Dhaliwal, the former CEO of CancerCare Manitoba, said this in a 2013 interview: 'I would like to emphasize that there is much that we individually and collectively can do to reduce the risk of cancer. Take exercise. There is new and emerging evidence that it can reduce the risk of developing cancer by 30%. Thirty percent! If we had a pill that did this, and it cost thousands of dollars, we'd all be screaming for that pill. And yet, it is something that is within our control.' So you see, exercise is an example of something that is virtually without cost and would have a huge impact on reducing the number of cancer diagnoses we see every year, especially in North America."

"So I should start to exercise daily—and that's all I need to do?"

"Well, no, there are a lot of other factors to consider, but it would certainly be a great start. Know that daily exercise has to be at least 30 minutes of vigorous activity, though. An active lifestyle is what's required. In fact, recent research shows that being sedentary for most of your day—even with that daily exercise—is as bad as not exercising at all and can actually counterbalance a great deal of the benefit that your daily half-hour of exercise provides you. So, you can get significant benefit from changing the way you work, even if you have a desk job."

"I don't understand. What's the difference between getting regular exercise and not being sedentary?"

"Well, you can get half an hour of vigorous exercise every day and still be at increased risk of cancer—and other health problems—if you spend the rest of your day sitting. So, it's recommended that you get up and walk for a few minutes every hour. If you have the flexibility at work, get a ball to sit on rather than a chair, or get a standing desk at which you can spend some of your desk time. Better yet, get a treadmill desk where you can walk while working."

"A treadmill desk?"

"Okay, that is probably not practical for most people, but the idea is that the more active you are—even if the activity is simply walking in place for a lot of your day—the better off you are in general, and the less likely it is you will get cancer."

"That's interesting. What are other environmental changes I can make to lessen my risk of cancer?"

"Let me give you my list, and then we can talk about it. Here are the general categories: activity, diet, alcohol, tobacco, and sunlight."

"Have we talked out the subject of activity already?"

"Almost. The general rules are three-fold. First, get 30 minutes of aerobic exercise each day—that's exercise where your heart rate and breathing are elevated but not where you feel exhausted—in the form of running, biking, swimming, or hiking. The key is to do exercise that you like, is fun for you, and will elevate your heart rate. Second, if you have a job where you sit a lot, take some time every hour to get up and walk around. I'd suggest five minutes per hour to take a walk down the hall or around the building. Third, try to incorporate activity into your lifestyle. Try biking to work or walking up the stairs rather than taking the elevator. Remember that this is not about weight loss or even fitness in the standard view of things; it's medicine, designed to keep you from getting cancer."

"Exercise as medicine. That's a radical idea."

"Yes, it's not the typical way we view medicine these days. But pills are not the only way to prevent or even cure disease."

"What about the other factors?"

"The next one is diet. That is not *a diet* as in calorie reduction. Talking about *dieting* is a bad way to discuss changing what you eat and how you approach food. I am not concerned about your calorie count per se or even your body mass index (BMI). I also do not have a vested interest in a specific kind of diet, not by name, anyway. It simply doesn't interest me what doctor or health guru has put his or her name onto a group of foods you are told to eat. What I'm interested in is a change in what you eat in order to ensure that your risk of cancer is as low as possible."

"So no fad diets, and no calorie counting. Got it."

"Right. Just as I am not interested in having you scientifically track the effects of your exercise, I am not interested in having you lose weight through dieting. I care about you putting the right set of foods into your mouth—your diet."

"What should my diet be then?"

"You won't be surprised when I tell you it should be balanced between the various food groups: dairy, fruits and vegetables, meats, grains, and oils. But that balance needs to lean towards fruits and vegetables—you can never eat too many fruits and vegetables—and away from meat and fat. I cannot tell you what the specific composition should be for you, but, if you stay away from processed foods (things that come pre-made in cans and packages), fatty meats (including what you find in fast food restaurants), and junk food (things with high fat, salt, and sugar content), you've made a good start."

"Okay. That makes two; what's next?"

"Let's tackle alcohol. As you know, alcohol is responsible for a whole host of societal ills. However, I'm not going to advocate abstinence, not only because it's not practical, but because I'm not sure it's particularly beneficial. Instead, what I'm going to promote is moderation. It's simple as that. Drink for enjoyment, not to get drunk. Feel free to drink regularly but not to excess. Have a glass of wine with your meal or a beer or two with your friends after work or on a hot day, but do not overdo it. Once again, I cannot tell you what is right for you, and there may be other issues at play that make it undesirable for you to drink at all. But the general principle is to use alcohol in moderation."

"I can live with that. What about tobacco?"

"Here's an irony. If a company came today to Health Canada or to the FDA in the United States and tried to get permission to sell tobacco products, it would be flatly denied. Tobacco, whether smoked or chewed, is a very bad substance. There is no way to overstate it. And while there are a lot of misconceptions about the direct causal links between tobacco and cancer, suffice it to say, you should avoid it. This is not one to take in moderation."

"What do you mean, misconceptions?"

"It's important to realize there isn't a direct one-to-one causal connection between smoking and cancer. That's why many people can point to someone, a brother or uncle or grandfather, who 'smoked a pack a day all his life and never got cancer.' This is falsely used as 'evidence' that smoking does not cause cancer. It's important that we deal with those real situations in order to dispel some myths about smoking and cancer."

"Alright. So, my grandfather smoked a lot, and he did not die of cancer. But you're saying that's not evidence that smoking is not bad for you."

"Correct. The first thing to note is that anecdotal evidence—
evidence based on stories—is not the best to hold up as proof of
anything. The second is that while smoking doesn't cause cancer in
everyone who smokes, it's a virtual certainty that if you do get lung or
mouth or tongue cancer and you smoke, it's the smoking that caused it
in you. Finally, smoking causes a whole host of other problems that can
harm your health or kill you, even if you don't get cancer."

"Hmmm, I see."

"What did your grandfather die of?"

"He had a stroke."

"Stroke is a major health breakdown which has also been closely
linked to smoking. So, it's quite possible that your grandfather still died
from complications related to smoking."

"Wow, I've never thought of it that way. But isn't it the case that,
after a certain point in your life, it doesn't make any difference if you
quit or not?"

"Not at all. Quitting will always be helpful both to extend your life
as well as increase its quality. It's never too late to quit smoking, and
it's always too early to begin. ... As for the fifth lifestyle factor you can
control, that's perhaps the hardest one these days: exposure to sunlight."

"Sigh. I love the sun. Where we live, summer seems so short, and, in
winter, the days themselves are so short that I relish every moment I can
spend in the sun."

"I hear you, and that's one reason talking about limiting your
exposure to the sun is so hard. That, and the years of media that have
told you a bronzed complexion is sexy and healthy."

"Everyone wants that lifeguard tan, right?"

"Right, but it's killing people every year. Over 82,000 people will
get skin cancer in Canada in 2014, and the vast majority of these are
caused by exposure to the sun or to UV rays in indoor tanning beds.
Let me quote from the 2014 report from Health Canada: 'Skin cancer
is the most common cancer in Canada, with an estimated 6,500 new
cases of cutaneous malignant melanoma (hereafter called melanoma)
and 76,100 cases of non-melanoma skin cancer (NMSC) expected to be
diagnosed in 2014 ... . Together melanoma and NMSC will account for
nearly the same number of new cancer cases as the four major cancers
combined (lung, breast, colorectal, prostate).'"

"Wow, that's a lot! Unbelievable that there's that much skin cancer!
What can I do to reduce my chances of getting it?"

"You need to protect yourself from the direct effects of exposure to the sun, and that's true regardless of the colour of your skin. While people of African descent don't get skin cancers as often as Caucasians, when they do get it, it tends to be far more serious because it goes undetected for much longer. Adequate protection means using sunscreen with at least SPF 15 any time you're out in the sun—and stay out of the sun altogether during peak UV periods, between 10:00 a.m. and 3:00 p.m. Wear a hat to protect your head, and, finally, never use tanning beds, ever!"

"But can't I just get a base tan before I start exposing myself to the sun? Won't that protect me?"

"No, I'm afraid not. Any change in colour to your skin means damage, and any damage can lead to skin cancer, not to mention premature aging of your skin, the largest organ of your body. We've got to get it into our heads that the colour we were born is the colour we ought to stay. At least that's something people knew in Victorian times, when they tried very hard to protect their complexions from the sun."

"So, I can reduce my risk of cancer by changing my lifestyle: exercise, diet, alcohol, tobacco, and sun exposure?"

"That's right."

"But what about tests? Can't doctors do tests on me to catch cancer early?"

"Yes, to some extent. And early detection is good because it ensures that you get the best possible outcome. But even better than relying on medical tests is taking responsibility for yourself. You can do a lot to ensure cancer is caught early or doesn't even develop at all."

"How do I do that?"

"Well, you have to start with knowing your body, your family history, and your risk factors. Armed with that, you can look for changes and be aware of the kinds of disease that people in your family and people of your age and ethnicity tend to get. Then work with your family doctor to ensure that new things get caught before they become real problems."

"Can you expand on those three things? Body, history, and risk?"

"Sure. Let's start with your body. You know you. You've lived with your body all your life. You know whether a certain pain is something you get all the time or whether it's new. You know when a condition has been caused by an specific event—my leg hurts because I fell down—or whether the cause is unknown. You can tell whether that lump you feel in your breast tissue or on your testicle is new, or whether that's just the way it's always been. And you know whether that feeling of being really tired all the time is because you're running 30 kilometres a day, or whether you're getting winded just walking up a flight of stairs."

"Yes, I need to pay attention to what my body is telling me."

"That's right. You are the best judge of that. And beyond that, you can also consult with friends, family, and your spouse. Ask them whether they've noticed anything different about your appearance, or whether they've heard you complain about anything new. Because, frankly, sometimes you can miss things that are plain to others."

"And if I find something, then what?"

"Well, go see your doctor, and move on from there."

"What about family history? How does that come into play?"

"Family history is critical to create a good surveillance plan for cancers—well, for all disease, really. Some cancer predispositions are inherited, so if there is a lot of cancer in your family, you might be at higher risk genetically. Or some cancer may just 'run in your family' because you all live and work in the same environment, for example. By knowing what kinds of cancers your relatives have (or have had) and at what age they got them, you can help your family doctor determine when it's prudent to start intensive surveillance. As an example, the standard time to start surveillance for colon cancer is at age 50. However, if either of your parents or any of your siblings has had colon cancer, it's recommended that you have a colonoscopy 10 years before the age your relative got it—or at 40, whichever is earlier. So, if your mom got colon cancer at the age of 45, your siblings and you should have a scope at age 35. And, if it's determined that your mom has an inherited cancer syndrome, such as Lynch, it may be recommended that you start getting scopes as early as 20."

"Will all family doctors know this stuff?"

"Not necessarily. There are guidelines, but no one doctor will be on top of everything with the massive amount of information out there today. It's good for you to ask questions of your doctor and help him help you in the best possible way."

"Are there other risk factors besides my family history?"

"Sure, there is environmental risk, risk from age, and risk from ethnicity. Environmental risk may be from your current environment, or it could be from past exposures to things. For example, if you'd worked in a coal mine when you were in your 20s, you'd be at increased risk for lung cancer. If you were a mechanic and had been exposed to asbestos dust in older brakes, you'd be at increased risk for lung cancer. Had you been in the area of the Chernobyl or Fukushima nuclear disasters, you'd be at risk of certain cancers. And if you lived in an area where radon gas accumulated naturally in the basement of your home, you'd be at increased risk of lung cancer. If you'd ever had radiation treatment for a cancer in the past, you could have an increased risk of another cancer in the same area. None of that is to say you would get cancer, but all of those situations would be risk factors that you and your family doctor would need to recognize. Increased risk doesn't mean you're going to get cancer. What it does mean is that there's a larger statistical likelihood that you'll get cancer over somebody else with the same lifestyle and DNA as you but who hasn't been exposed to the same things."

"That's an awful lot to keep track of!"

"Yes, it is, but it needs to be done because the more you know, the more you can do to ensure the best outcome."

"What about age?"

"Cancer generally results from the accumulation of errors in a cell's DNA, so the older you are, the greater the accumulation. Also, the older you get, the more errors your cells make, so it stands to reason that your likelihood of getting cancer increases as you age. One of the downsides of modern technology increasing our average life span is that we actually grow old enough to get diseases that were not as common one or two hundred years ago. Early humans rarely got cancer because most of them died by the time they were 40."

"I guess I need to be more vigilant about my health as I get older."

"Yes. That's why it's recommended that people get regular colon, breast, and prostate exams as they age. However, there are downsides to this hyper-vigilance as well. You see, as we age, the treatment for these things sometimes becomes more harmful than the disease itself."

"Really?"

"Sure. Prostate cancer is an excellent example. While prostate cancer cannot be dismissed as a benign disease because 35,000 men in North America die from it every year, there are many men who receive very invasive and life-altering treatments who would not have suffered any ill effects from having the disease progress. Left alone, many prostate cancers would not progress far enough to do significant harm until very old age, if ever.

"Breast cancer is another example where hyper-vigilant attitudes have been exposed as counterproductive. The prevailing wisdom about aggressive screening regimes and radical surgeries has been changing as more information is amassed about how ineffective some of the treatments and practices have been."

"I had never realized that. ... So how does ethnicity enter into this discussion?"

"Well, ethnicity implies some commonality of genetics. As we've discussed, your genetics combine with your environment to provide either resistance or susceptibility to cancer. As a result, it stands to reason that certain ethnic groups would be more prone to certain kinds of cancers because they share both genetics and, oftentimes, . environment. However, the discussion of ethnicity and cancer is not as simple as being able to connect certain cultural groups with certain cancers because there are also socio-economic factors that relate to survivability."

"Can you give me an example?"

"In North America, women of African, Aboriginal, and Hispanic descent tend to have a lower survival rate from breast cancer than do Caucasian women. However, this has nothing to do with their genetics or ethnicity and everything to do with their average socio-economic status. Women in all three of these groups tend not to have family physicians; therefore, they get diagnosed at more advanced stages of cancer than do women who get care from a physician they see regularly."

"Well, thanks for all the light you've shed on cancer for me. I really didn't know there were so many things to think about when considering cancer prevention. All those risk factors I can control, and the additional surveillance I need to seek out as I age ... ."

"You're very welcome. Cancer can be beaten, and the best way to do that is to not get it in the first place."

38

I Talk About Heritable Cancer Syndromes

"Very strange things comes to our knowledge in families, miss; bless your heart, what you would think to be phenomenons, quite. ... Aye, and even in gen-teel families, in high families, in great families ... you have no idea ... what games goes on!"

Mr. Bucket to Volumnia in Charles Dickens, *Bleak House*

As a carrier of a genetic mutation that predisposes me to cancer, I have a special interest in advocating for the best solutions to determine who is at risk and how surveillance is best conducted. In the best possible world, we would all know our genetic status and whether we carried any harmful mutations, we'd get appropriate surveillance to ensure that any ill effects were caught as early as possible, and, of course, the knowledge of any genetic mutation wouldn't adversely affect us, whether psychologically, in finding employment, or in getting insurance. However, as I've previously remarked, this is not a perfect world. Genetic testing is expensive, and it has the potential not only to unsettle people psychologically, but also to threaten their financial well-being, through possible difficulty in getting health or life insurance, for instance.

Knowledge is power, however; in this case, it's the power to advocate for proper surveillance for your family and yourself. It also prompts society to wrestle with questions about the relative cost and benefit of preventing people from getting sick to treating them when the medical, personal, and social costs are at their highest. I'm a practical guy, and I think we can find the compromises that would allow us to spend an appropriate amount of money to determine the genetic status of people who are most at risk and then work to keep them, as much as possible, from getting sick. Therefore, we should provide simple ways to allow people to evaluate their own risk factors, present any concerns to their doctors, and, when warranted, have access to genetic testing in order to determine their status. Once that happens, at-risk family groups can be identified, and further testing and surveillance can be targeted.

I'd like to provide some simple diagnostic questions here to help you determine whether or not you should be asking your doctor about genetics and cancer. These are general and will only help steer you in a certain direction. There may be doctors who think this is a bad idea because they will be inundated with questions about genetics and testing, but I think the benefit of increasing the visibility of genetic heredity as a cause for cancer far outweighs any problems that might be caused by too many people asking too many questions—if that is even possible.

To make things clear, I need to establish context: you must have access to general medical knowledge about your biological family. It will require careful, thorough research to collect the critical information, but this is an important task well worth your time. There may also be a significant emotional cost to do this, particularly if you are separated from your biological relatives—if you are adopted, for example, or estranged from your family. Without access to your biological family, however, the only questions you can answer will be those about you and your own experience with cancer.

Questions About You

These questions are about you and establish risk based on your personal experience with cancer.

1) Have you had cancer? If you have, further questions will help determine whether you are part of a discernible pattern. If you answered, "Yes," go to the next question. Otherwise, skip it and jump directly to the next section.

2) Did you have cancer between the ages of 18 and 50? This would establish that you've had an adult cancer, but that you got it at a young age. If you were younger than 18 and got cancer, you had a childhood cancer: cancers which occur in children often have different causes than those which occur in adults and, as a result, are often disregarded in these kinds of questionnaires. Nevertheless, if you did have a childhood cancer, answers to the following questions may could still help reveal a pattern in your family.

Questions About Your Immediate Family

Your immediate family (sometimes called your first-degree relatives) are people connected to you by only one line on your family tree. They include your biological parents, siblings, and children.

1) Has one or more of your first-degree relatives had cancer between the ages of 18 and 50?

2) If you collect your first-degree relatives together (including yourself), has there been more than one occurrence of cancer, and were those cancers similar? This question requires clarification. Firstly, if one of your first-degree relatives had two or more cancers which seemed to be unrelated, that counts as yes to this question. Secondly, the word similar is more of a challenge to clarify. Certain genetic syndromes create cancers in many different organs that, by virtue of belonging to the same syndrome, could be called similar. The BRCA mutation, for instance, has been linked to breast and colon cancer, so those trends would be important to spot. On the other hand, the Lynch syndrome set of related cancers would include colon, uterine, bladder, and other cancers. Thus, the best approach would be to note all cancers and the person's age at onset of the cancer and then, together with your doctor, do some research to find out whether the different kinds of cancer could actually be related or not.

Questions About Your Extended Family

For the sake of this discussion, your extended family is everyone in your family tree who falls under your grandparents or their siblings and who is connected biologically (genetically) to you. For example, your dad's brother would be included, as would your cousins, but your aunt (the woman who married your dad's brother) would not. Neither would any people who have joined your family through marriage or adoption. For some people, extended family can include a very large number of people, but if you are able to get this medical information for them, you will be well positioned to detect heritable patterns that are as important for them as they are for you.

1)   Have two or more members of your extended family had cancer between the ages of 18 and 50?

2)   Have these cancers been similar?

The preceding questions have been as much about simple encouragement to take a close look at your family tree for incidents of cancer as it has been about providing you with a screening test. When I had my first cancer, I was oblivious of the prevalence of cancer in my family, so when my doctors asked me about it, I answered incorrectly: "My mother had uterine cancer but no one else that I can think of." However, as I now study my family tree, I can see that a great deal more information was available then, had I only known.

If, as you look back over your answers to these six questions, you see a lot of people with similar kinds of cancer, especially in middle age or even younger adult years, that is a good indicator a genetic factor is at work. If so, you should take this information (the family tree with cancers and age of onset marked on it) to your doctor and ask about the appropriateness of genetic counselling and, after that, genetic testing.

Should you see patterns of cancer, there are two things you ought to expect and, if necessary, advocate for. The first is genetic counselling. This happens before any genetic testing gets done, allowing a professional with knowledge of genetic syndromes to judge whether your suspicions actually show sufficient evidence to be of serious concern. If warranted, depending on the types and pervasiveness of cancers in your family tree, the genetics professional would recommend genetic testing for possible mutations. In addition, the professional would review the implications of testing for you and other members of your family, especially your children (whether children already born or those you might have in the future).

Genetic testing is done using a sample of blood taken at a doctor's office or a medical lab. The blood sample is small and the procedure relatively painless (more than a mosquito bite but less than skinning your knee). This sample is sent to a lab, and, in a matter of days, weeks, or months, the results are sent back, indicating what kind of mutation you have, if any. Whether testing positive or negative, you would discuss the results with the genetic counsellor or a geneticist. From there, any course of surveillance necessary for you would be established.

I conclude by reasserting: knowledge is power. Some might say it is better not to know. Respectfully, I disagree with that sentiment. Many beneficial things can be done to reduce the potentially harmful effects of a genetic mutation, even to the point of preventing cancers that could otherwise arise. However, you cannot watch for something that you do not know might be ahead.

A Final Word

When I started this book, I intended to recount a set of events in hope that the experiences I have had and the lessons I have learned would be of interest and help to others.

For me, this experience has been so much more than that. It has been a journal of much of my life, some of which was perhaps 20 years overdue. It has been a prompter to memory. But most of all, it has been a reaffirmation of the power of community. This community, my community, saw me through my darkest hours and upheld me in more ways than can be counted or recounted.

While these are the final words in this book, they are not the final words in my story—a story that I hope will end many years hence. Above all, a story that will be full of life, no matter its length.

A Note from the Author

It has been almost a year since I received my first copy of *What I Learned from Cancer*. And what a ride it's been. I've learned a lot about writing and publishing and how independently produced books get out into the world. One of the themes in this book is that of community, and I've learned that community is the determining factor in the success of any book and especially independent ones.

So, if you enjoyed this book and you think that other people would benefit from reading it, you can help out. Do one (or all) of the following:

- Go to Amazon.com, find this book, and post a review. If you are not in the USA, you can also post that review on your country specific Amazon site: reviews are not shared between the various Amazon sites.
- Go to Goodreads, and post the same review that you posted on Amazon.
- Take a picture of yourself with the book and post it on your Facebook feed and tell people that it is great and you recommend they read it.
- Tweet that same picture to your followers. Hashtags could include #cancer, #hereditarycancer, #WhatILearnedFromCancer, etc.
- Don't forget about Instagram, Pinterest—wherever your social media platforms are.
- Encourage your local library to purchase a copy (or a hundred).
- Have your book club read the book. If you don't belong to one, join or start one. You can purchase the Book Club Bundle (10 paperbacks for the price of 9) at the Prompters to Life website (http://prompterstolife.com/shoppers) and I will visit your book club to tell stories and answer questions. If you live in Winnipeg—or somewhere that you'd be willing to take care of my travel expenses—I would be happy to come to your living room or wherever else you meet and be with your group. If you live further afield, I would be happy to visit via Skype or other video conferencing to anywhere in the world that the Internet reaches.

- Look for updates on my Facebook page, "Prompters to Life," and follow me on Twitter: @prompters.

Here are some links that you might find helpful, whether for yourself or to share:

- http://prompterstolife.com/shoppers — where you can purchase another copy of the book if you can't find it in a local book store.
- http://payhip.com/prompterstolife — where you can get a copy of the eBook, whether Kindle or Kobo/iBook.
- http://dennismaione.com — where you can find out all things "Dennis Maione," including upcoming events, current book projects, blogs, videos, and all of the services that I offer.

Dennis Maione
August 24th, 2015